"I can think of no better person than Jessica Kisiel to write the definitive book on how to move beyond the injury-pain cycle. Having overcome her own debilitating injuries and coached so many others to do the same, she has moved to the forefront of leaders in the field of body-mind healing. If you're ready to reclaim your body and life, I highly recommend this book."

Sonia Sommer
Structural Integration Practitioner and Soul Healer

D1496747

"Wow. This is a beautiful and powerful book with incredible wisdom to be gained. I'm only at the very beginning of my recovery journey, and yet I have already come so far in just three months. And, it's not just from a physical point of view. It's been 17 years since I broke my hip, and I have many bad body compensations, but I do believe I will get there. And a lot of that belief is thanks to you, Jessica!"

Sasha MacSween
Chief Financial Officer (CFO), mother, elite swimmer and amateur cyclist

"Watching Jessica's journey from a high-performing athlete, to a struggling athlete plagued with injuries, then back to a high-performing athlete has been a pleasure and a delight. When she started her journey with Egoscue®, I saw someone worn down by injuries with little hope. BUT as she began her healing journey, the glimmer in her eye began to emerge, and little by little that developed into the fire in her belly. You know, the one you see in Athletes in pursuit. It came back!

Yet she wasn't content there. Instead she became an 'evangelist' for the Egoscue Method®, wanting to rescue other athletes from that nagging question that causes them to think . . . 'Was that my career ending injury?' 'Am I done?' Now she has brought her hope to you in written form. Both simple and powerful. Read on. You won't be disappointed."

John Cattermole
Master Egoscue [R] *Therapist (Clinic Director Egoscue* [R] *Phoenix)*

"Jessica takes readers on a down to earth, enlightening journey through the challenging world of athletic injuries and/or setbacks. This is an eloquent book, full of insights and practical information that transcends pain and loss – and becomes an inspiration."

Lisa Smole, BS, MBA
Certified Medical Support Clinical Hypnotherapist (CMS-CHt)
Fellow of the International Board of Hypnotherapy (FIBH)

"As a chiropractor, I work with people in chronic pain daily. I believe in the value of educating my patients about proper posture alignment and conditioning the deep postural muscles as a foundation for well-being. I am grateful to be able to refer my patients to a coach such as Jessica, as well as having this book as a helpful reference."

Nancy Savoia
Doctor of Chiropractic (DC)

"Jessica's teachings and exercises on alignment have been successful and essential in eliminating the recurring back spasms and hip discomfort that limited my training for years. I have been free of those problems for a few years now, and, as a result, I am increasing my training with a goal of completing an *Ironman Triathlon* when I am 70!"

Matt Briggs
Physicist, baritone sax player, triathlete

"The yoga tradition is based on the philosophy that the body, mind and spirit cannot be separated. *Winning the Injury Game* applies this vital principle to healing and athletics. Jessica expertly demonstrates how treating an injury, or training for a sport, is most effective when consideration is given to the physical, mental, emotional and spiritual states of the athlete."

Mike Hoog
Physical Therapist

"*Winning the Injury Game* promotes a holistic approach to healing and challenges us to think differently about how we care for our injuries and chronic pain. Using her story of recovery, Jessica shares valuable insights that will benefit and inspire anyone who is struggling with an injury and who has not responded to traditional medical treatment."

Susan Grubb
Doctor of Oriental Medicine (DOM)
Licensed Massage Therapist (LMT)
Licensed Acupuncturist

"*Winning the Injury Game* is one of the most insightful texts for athletic performance and athletic durability that has been published in years. Jessica Kisiel's thorough analysis of the most innovative and diverse scientific approaches towards biomechanics and human performance makes this a treasure trove of knowledge that will benefit Athletes and Rehabilitation Professionals alike. The book is clearly the result of years of study and discovery, laid out in a concise and easy-to-understand manner. *Winning the Injury Game* provides the Athlete Reader a pathway to fully understand their body and its ability for pain-free movement. Jessica utilizes personal experience in a way that will provide understanding and hope to the reader, but avoids becoming an anecdotal self-help journal. Complex biomechanical, physiological, emotional, and anatomical concepts are explained in easy-to-understand language with excellent examples and exercises. I will be recommending and making this book available to all of my patients."

"This book makes the mantra 'train smarter, not harder' truly possible!"

Raulan Young, MPT, PRC
Physical Therapist
Biomechanical Consultant
Owner of Proactive Physical Therapy, Idaho a Postural Restoration® Center

"As a voracious reader, I am always drawn to non-fictional books, articles, journals, and literary essays that offer a personal perspective based on personal experience. Jess Kisiel has been a student and patient whom I have always had a great deal of respect for because of her commitment to herself and her body. Her pedagogical process of imparting what she has experienced, discovered and practiced also helped her recover, heal and nurture her need to understand how to rely on and trust herself. I have watched her over the years discover herself and the process that best aligned and balanced her mind and body and their performance with each other. As therapeutic as this book's recommendations are, so are her personal accounts of the interconnections and patterned relationships of forces that reject healing and recovery. An example of these reflections and realizations are outlined in every chapter. Overall balance requires respect for the lungs and posture; and overall awareness of success requires respect for sensate awareness. She brings these concepts to realization, no matter what an individual is limited in or at. This book will help the reader enjoy finding true accountability in recovery, through a process that requires an alternative process of injury prevention that ultimately leads to a reduction of pain.

Game on!"

Ron Hruska MPA, PT
Executive Director
Postural Restoration Institute®

WINNING THE INJURY GAME

WINNING
THE INJURY GAME

Alignment Strategies for Healing and Performance

Jessica Kisiel, MS

Winning the Injury Game
Alignment Strategies for Healing and Performance

Editing by Whitney Pomeroy
Cover and author photo by Robert Villegas
Illustrations by Donovan Heimer
Book design and layout by Elena Perez

Printed in the United States of America.

Published by The Pain Free Athlete LLC in Moab, Utah.

The Pain Free Athlete

Stay in the game for life

www.thepfathlete.com

Library of Congress Cataloging-in-Publication Data
ISBN 978-0-9994425-0-0

This book is not intended as a substitute for the medical advice of physicians. The reader should regularly consult a physician in matters relating to his/her health and particularly with respect to any symptoms that may require diagnosis or medical attention. The information in this book is meant to supplement, not replace, proper sports training. Sports involving speed, equipment, balance and environmental factors pose some inherent risks. Readers are advised to take full responsibility for their safety and know their limits.

To my husband, Ken,
whose love and support
made this book possible.

Sections

mind

body

training

Table of Contents

3

How Your Mind Responds to Injury **43**

4

Seven Tips for Your Healing Journey **65**

5

Treating Your Injury **87**

6

7

11

Gaining Sensory Awareness 217

12

Developing Functional Strength 249

13

Wholistic Sports Training **277**

14

Seven Strategies for Sports Performance **301**

List of Illustrations

11

12

13

Foreword

*I*n *Winning the Injury Game*, Jessica Kisiel has taken a very complex subject, dissected all of the components, and presented practical and realistic solutions that simply work. One glance at the Table of Contents will reveal the in-depth subject matter, confirming that this book is not only a must-read but a must-do for athletes of any age, at all levels of performance and competition. In reality, it will greatly benefit every person with a need to solve his or her own problems with chronic pain and physical dysfunction.

One of the most important concerns for competitive athletes is how to preserve their bodies for physical function and performance for the long haul, while simultaneously being cautious about sacrificing their bodies ultimately to win the trophy, even in the face of suffering through pain and chronic recurrent injuries. If you have wondered why you are not recovering from your injury, chronic recurrent pain or compound injuries, and if you are not responding to standard treatment protocols, this book will help you discover answers you may have never considered in regard to proper muscle recruitment, skeletal alignment, static posture and posture in motion. Have you been wondering what is taking you out of the game and how you can get back into it and healthy again? I believe that *Winning the Injury Game* will help you solve the puzzle. Conversely, you may be in great pain-free condition and want to take yourself to a higher level of performance. The principles in this book will help get you there.

Winning the Injury Game is one of the best and most comprehensive presentations of our time. It is clear, well-documented, and superbly referenced. Jessica has done some major thinking out of the box in order to energize our thinking about how to put our healing processes into practice. She has merged some of the most important modern-day works that are based on the principles of the Egoscue Method®—for postural correction through proper form and function—and the Postural Restoration Institute®—for core cylinder of strength (the all-important breathing mechanism) and how it affects the rest of body function. Other major authors and contributions are included to provide a balanced approach and address the areas of proper musculoskeletal function, alignment, and balance. The book is outlined with clear illustrations, making a difficult subject easy to understand. And while there are many good books written on the subject of pain-relief and healing that address fragmented treatments of the human body, Jessica has done a wonderful job in concluding how physical, mental, spiritual and emotional realms all contribute to recovery and wellness. In this book, you will discover unconventional answers to both common and unusual injury problems based on genuine principles of anatomical function and biomechanical physics that are nicely demonstrated, documented and cross-referenced. Using these principles, Jessica explains how to stay in the game, no matter what the sport, and how to do it right.

Winning the Injury Game is a guide to your success, not a doctrine, which helps not only the athlete but all individuals make intelligent decisions based on applied functional anatomy and kinetic science, providing real solutions. As you read through the pages, you will discover new horizons for yourself and will probably come to realize that you can become your own miracle (and that age is no limitation of accomplishing your goals). You will read and relate to Jessica's internal and external struggles as she tried to find important answers for managing injuries and related issues. She is candidly frank about her own injuries and the confusion that set in as she sought standard treatment options. I think each of us can identify with her story and other examples provided in the book. I know I can.

Since junior high school and over the years, I have endeavored to stay in good fitness through strength and aerobic training plus a variety of sports, horse activities such as endurance competition and horse packing, hunting and fishing, backpacking and golf. Having participated in all of these sports, and having ridden thousands of miles on horseback, I have had my share of injuries. Specific exercise regimens (that sometimes took one or two years for maximum recovery) put me back in action, but when I discovered the Egoscue Method® of postural correction and maintenance through proper motion and exercise over 12 years ago, my understanding of physical health jumped to an entirely new level. It also gave me more confidence and better conditioning/fitness. It became a whole new learning and training experience. This is also augmented by other components, as outlined in Jessica's book. Consequently, I do not miss a day of performing a wide variety of postural exercises and fitness workouts, and I continue to use the posture principles as the foundation for all activities of daily life, work, sports, recreation and other conditioning programs. At age 75 I am able to carry a full golf bag on any arduous golf course (18+ holes) while shooting a single-digit handicap score, and I can still backpack 60+ pounds in the Rocky Mountains. Having better alignment and balance means being able to move with less effort, applying power with less force, and coordinating movements with more positive results. I believe in these fundamental principles so strongly that when my two sports-loving grandsons were ages 6 and 10, I started them on daily postural and natural strength routines to prevent injuries and enhance their athletic talents. I believe that God has created each of us in unique ways, and that it is our responsibility to care for ourselves appropriately so that we can remain healthy, pain-free, and in turn, be of good service to others.

Every individual is different, and every situation is different. It is important to take responsibility for yourself to get well and stay well. This is not a quick fix. Once you get it, though, it will definitely be a life-changing experience. The ultimate outcome will be superb physical fitness and conditioning, pain-free movement, enhanced soundness in body and mind, improved athletic abilities, and greater joy and satisfaction in sports and life. Jessica outlines the path to achieve these results in her Wheel of Sports Performance.

It is my understanding that Jessica has taken nine years of perseverance to write about this crucial subject through challenging personal trials and a great deal of research. I would consider this book a mini-masterpiece. This work is so important that it should be studied and read by all physicians, athletes, coaches, trainers, therapists, workmen's compensation boards, and personal injury attorneys—as well as the average person trying to understand and maintain sound structural health.

Are you going to cross the finish line in good condition? This book will explain how you can accomplish your goals and stay the course. Be patient, be persistent, and be committed. Think out of the box. You will overcome and succeed. Most of all, have fun as you learn how your anatomy works. Take on the challenge, and find out that you can heal your pain.

Michael L. Rothman, M.D.
Santa Fe, New Mexico

Fellow American Academy Orthopaedic Surgeons, Emeritus
Fellow International Academy of Independent Medical Examiners
Fellow American College of Forensic Examiners
Postural Alignment Specialist (PAS) and Advanced Exercise Therapist (AET), Egoscue University® Certified
Member, American College of Sports Medicine
New Mexico Medical Society and Orthopaedic Society
Active PAS and AET Practice

Proverbs 3:5-6 *Trust in the Lord with all your heart + lean not on your own understanding. In all your ways submit to him + he will make your paths straight.*

Job 12:10 *In His hand is the life of every creature + breath of all mankind*

Hebrews 12:11-13

Philippians 4:13 *I can do all things through HIM who strengthens me*

Psalm 30:2 *Lord, My God, I called out to you for help + you healed me*

No discipline seems pleasant at the time but painful. Later on however it produces a harvest of righteousness and peace for those who have been trained by it.

Acknowledgments

Self-publishing this book was a huge yet greatly rewarding undertaking. I really didn't know what I was getting myself into when I started this project. I was compelled to share my message with others and was fortunate to find people who shared my passion for the material. I could not have completed this book without them.

I'll start from the beginning with two extraordinary individuals who volunteered their time to go over the early versions of the manuscript with me page by page—more than once! My sincere thanks to Jaqueline Kiplinger and Sandra West, whose contributions elevated the content and flow of the pages that follow. I also want to recognize my other content editors—Nancy Savoia, Lisa Smole, Gretchen Selby, and my writing coach, Rose Muenker—who each brought a different perspective and valuable insights. After all this input, it is with much gratitude that I acknowledge my copy editor and proofreader, Whitney Pomeroy, whose excellent skills greatly improved the ease of reading this sometimes technical material. She evaluated every word, hyphen, comma, and more. Her efforts make the text truly elegant.

The images you'll see in this book are awesome, making the information clear and straightforward. I was fortunate to be introduced to a highly gifted illustrator, Donovan Heimer. His patience was evident with every revision of an image, especially when I'd go back and decide to use his original drawing after trying several changes.

Covers sell books, and I think this one is superb, thanks to the talents of my photographer and graphic designer, Robert Villegas. I have had a vision in my mind of what I wanted ever since I rode the White Rim trail with my husband many years ago, and Robert brilliantly brought it to life. Conveniently, I had recently moved to Moab, Utah; Robert was visiting the Canyonlands area, one of his favorite places to explore archeology, and while he was there, he masterfully took the photo that became the cover.

Initially, I thought I'd do the layout of the book myself since I'd had some experience with similar software. However, sitting with my layout designer, Elena Perez, and watching her masterfully manipulate the computer application (with much better grace and composure than I would have demonstrated) reassured me that I had made the right decision in engaging her assistance. Most of the stylistic touches that add class to this book were her ideas.

I am eternally grateful for the dedication and assistance of all of these wonderful people. But this book wouldn't be a success without you, the reader. You are the one whom I appreciate the very most. With all the books to choose from, you selected mine. I am so pleased and humbled, hoping that what follows will provide you with thoughtful and inspiring information that positively and powerfully impacts your life.

Introduction

*M*any people believe that injuries are inevitable when you play sports. Some are also under the assumption that the longer you play, the more pain you will endure. Although some injuries are the result of "accidents" and are out of your control—a skier slamming into you on the slopes, a teammate falling on your ankle, or a car hitting you while you're riding your bicycle—other injuries are more predictable. These foreseeable injuries come on slowly. They also have warning signs, such as that nagging pain in your elbow that steadily becomes worse, eventually forcing you to stop playing tennis, golf, or throwing sports. I believe this second type of injury is preventable. With proper preparation and training, you can avoid these gradually-occurring injuries that could linger for weeks, months, and even years. I will explain how in this book.

Most likely, however, you picked up this book because you hurt—NOW. Prevention sounds like a good long-term strategy, but first, you need relief from your current, relentless pain. Let me assure you, this is not the end of your sports. *You will play again!* I know you are suffering right now. You just want to feel better and get back to life as usual. I empathize with your fears about being able to fully heal and regain your athletic lifestyle. I understand that being active is a big part of who you are and what you love to do for fun. Athletics is what makes you feel alive, happy, and good about yourself. It keeps you sane. *I get it!* And I recognize that not being able to play sports is devastating to your life in so many ways.

I've been there, more times than I care to remember. Over a span of eight years, I had a joint surgery every other year: 2001 (left knee), 2003 (left knee), 2005 (left knee), and 2007 (left hip). I didn't know if this cycle was ever going to stop, or if my body was just going to continue to deteriorate, bringing an end to my athletics—forever. My full story is explained in the first chapter of this book, but in a nutshell, I was miserable. I didn't know what to do or where to turn for help. And I don't want you to feel that way. This is why I wrote this book. I want to guide you on your healing

1

journey so it can be shorter and easier for you than it was for me. This book is written from two perspectives: through my eyes as an injured athletic patient in chronic pain, and through my viewpoint as a coach for others. It is a collection of the lessons that I have learned through my personal healing and that my clients have taught me as I supported them in their recovery. My intention is to help you avoid the mistakes I made and, instead, to learn from my athletic experience and professional knowledge.

Winning the Injury Game is written for the athlete who is hurting right now. It is for the active person whose pain persists, despite repeated treatments. This book is for the sports enthusiast who realizes that the standard approach to healing an injury isn't working; this enthusiast is open to new ideas and a holistic approach to recovery. This book is for anyone who wants to be active for life. It is for the person who appreciates that treating what seems to be a musculoskeletal injury is often the result of imbalances throughout several body systems. This last point is one of the key discoveries I made in my recovery process, and it is an underlying premise of this book.

First, I want to be clear: this book is about chronic physical pain. I have inserted the word "physical" between "chronic" and "pain" to specify that I am talking about damage to the body itself. We can also suffer "chronic pain" derived from mental and emotional causes, which will also be discussed in this book. However, when I use the phrase "chronic pain," I am generally referring to the physical aspect.

Chronic pain is the longstanding pain that doesn't go away. It is not the result of an acute accident or broken bone; it comes on slowly, gradually getting worse over time. Chronic pain often doesn't have a well-defined cause, which can make it difficult to diagnose and treat. Chronic pain is often the result of microtraumas, as described by Gray Cook, MSPT, OCS, CSCS, leading physical therapist and creator of the *Functional Movement Screen (FMS)*: "Microtrauma results from small amounts of stress imposed on the body over time caused by poor biomechanics and overtraining."[1] I'll add that this physical stress, which is the result of misdirected forces through our tissues and joints when we move,[2] is often due to skeletal misalignments. This is why chronic pain comes on slowly, why it tends to happen when we're older, and why chronic pain usually doesn't go away on its own: it is an accumulation of damage, or "microtraumas," that we've had our whole life to develop. As Cook states, "poor biomechanics" are a cause of microtrauma.[1] Biomechanics often do not improve without re-training. Of course, when we're injured, we change our biomechanics, such as limping when we twist our ankle, but this alters our movements negatively and contributes to the accumulation of damage within our body. The longer we have been out of balance, the longer the pain persists, and the stronger and more deeply wired these unhealthy movement patterns become. The consistent pain we feel is frequently a symptom of our body's asymmetries. You'll learn much more about structural alignment, symptoms and causes of pain in Chapters 5-8.

Now that we're on the same page, I'll reiterate my point: chronic pain represents an imbalance in the body systems beyond the musculoskeletal. All of a body's systems work together and are dependent on one another to maintain a person's wellness. For example, when the bones of your skeleton are not aligned, you may develop symptoms within other body systems, like I did. I suffered from gastrointestinal (GI) distress, TMD (temporomandibular disorder), reproductive system issues, constipation, and ringing in my ears (tinnitus). Physical misalignment that can be seen from the outside impacts the position and function of the internal structures, such as organs, blood vessels, and ear canals. The body is a dynamic system, balanced through the exchange of pressures, air, gases, fluids, nutrients, and waste products, among other things. If the inner structures (or *tubes*)—intestines, esophagus, ureters—are kinked due to bony misalignments or tight tissue restrictions, then the precious substances within these tubes are not able to flow freely, creating pain and disorder within the body systems.[3] As an example, one of my clients with acid reflux was able to stop taking his little purple pill when his posture improved. By changing the alignment of his internal organs, fluids could move more smoothly throughout his body, and his symptoms were reduced.

Regulating the nervous system is particularly important in relation to healing and pain relief. There are two branches to our autonomic nervous system (ANS): the sympathetic nervous system (SNS), which elicits the "fight-or-flight" stress response, and the parasympathetic nervous system (PNS), which elicits the relaxation response.[4] These systems work in opposition to each other: when one is active, the other is inhibited (turned off). Our modern lives are full of stressors, causing many of us to be chronically stuck in a sympathetic state. Dr. Lissa Rankin, a physician leading the way for holistic health care, tells us that we have 50 or more stress responses a day. We cannot take advantage of our bodies' natural healing processes when we are in a sympathetic state. It is only when we relax that the body is able to heal. Relaxation is our natural state. In her book *Mind Over Medicine*, Dr. Rankin writes,

> When the relaxation response is induced, the parasympathetic nervous system is in charge. Only in this relaxed state can the body's natural self-repair mechanisms go about the business of repairing what gets out of whack in the body, the way the body is designed.[5]

As you will learn in this book, chronic activation of the stress response also affects your posture—from your foot position all the way to your head position. The breath is the gateway into your parasympathetic nervous system (PNS). Proper breathing mechanics and correct alignment of the respiratory system are essential for healing. Resilience, as brilliantly defined by Jocelyn Olivier, a visionary in the study of body somatics, is "the ability to move freely between sympathetic arousal and parasympathetic release."[6] This definition could also be used to describe the concept of "neutrality" from the Postural Restoration Institute® (PRI). Neutrality includes the ability to seamlessly switch between the sympathetic and parasympathetic nervous systems and to skillfully alternate between the left and right sides of the body and brain.[3] I will discuss this more in Chapters 10 and 11.

Lack of alignment (which causes pain in our physical structure and body systems) often reflects imbalances in the emotional, mental and spiritual aspects of our life. Please understand that I am not using the word *spiritual* in a religious context. My reference to *spiritual* is with regard to your character. Are you being authentic to who you are, what you believe, and what you value? Examples of being out of balance in these areas include some of the following issues: (1) emotionally—feeling depressed and unmotivated; (2) mentally—having confused and negative thinking; and (3) spiritually—failing to follow your calling or to live with purpose. As an example, at the time of my hip injury, I was in an unfulfilling job that was outside my area of expertise; it made me feel frustrated and inadequate daily. Beyond the work stress, my family relations were distant and strained. The only positives I had in my world were my friends, canine companions, and adoring husband, whose support kept me going.

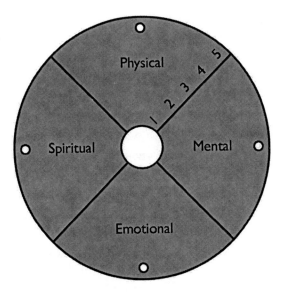

Figure i-1. Symmetry in these four dimensions is essential for healing and optimal performance.

After making many changes in my life, I heard some very wise words from my mentor in posture alignment therapy: he told me that each client who comes through our office door is out of balance in multiple areas of his or her life. That wisdom has proven to be so accurate with me and several of my clients. I need to look beyond the easily identifiable physical asymmetries and instead use my wellness coaching skills to recognize the imbalances in my client's cognitive state of being. To completely recover from injury, as well as to achieve ultimate sports and human performance, a person must have balance in four dimensions: physical, emotional, mental and spiritual. To emphasize this point, Figure i-1 shows the inner hub of my Wheel of Sports Performance, which will be discussed in Chapter 13.

Jim Loehr, Ed.D., world renowned sports psychologist, and Tony Schwartz, president and founder of *The Energy Project*, discuss how each of these life dimensions has an associated energy capacity in their article, "The Making of a Corporate Athlete."[7] It is the interplay between these dimensions, paired with adequate stress and recovery cycles, that allows us to reach our peak performance. When we are in "the zone" or experiencing "flow," as the peak performance state is often termed, we are in alignment in these four dimensions and can achieve the unimaginable.

I know all of this because I have lived it. I have been in pain for much of my athletic life, and I have had multiple injuries and joint surgeries. I tried to heal through standard medical approaches but found I was still in pain at the end of those treatments. I had a choice to make: reduce my activities, accept my doctor's prediction of an imminent hip replacement, and give up my athletic dreams, or find another way to heal. I was challenged to discover a path, at the time unknown to me, that would bring me back into balance—a path that would allow me to overcome my chronic pain, continue playing sports, and return to high-level competition.

It has been a journey, but I've found my way. There were many turns and detours along my path that I never would have expected. As depicted on the cover of this book, my road to healing was not a straight line. Rather, it was a twisting, switchbacking trail. I made steady forward progress on my climb to recovery by continuously pushing the pedals over and never giving up. At times I felt I might be going in the wrong direction, but I soon realized there was a reason and purpose for my route deviations. The side trips provided me with opportunities to gain perspective, learn and grow. My indirect path to recovery revealed new possibilities and complementary approaches for healing that I never would have considered otherwise.

I recovered, not just physically but in many other ways, which you will learn through the pages of this book. I can now say that I am a better person because of my injuries and as a result of going through my healing process. I hope that at the end of your journey, you can say the same about yourself. I'm pretty sure that's not how you feel about it now, and I completely understand. It took me years to find the meaning in my injury. When I was hurting with my hip pain, just after I'd gone through three knee surgeries, I made a conscious choice to make the most of the situation and vowed to help others through the process. That's when I started to write this book, nearly a decade ago.

In *Winning the Injury Game*, I'll share the key discoveries I made about healing, pain, the body, sports training, and life. I'll show you how I transitioned from continuously abusing and ignoring my body to respecting and caring for myself without sacrificing my joints or activities. In the pages that follow, I'll take you on a journey from your current pain through healing in all the alignment dimensions so that you can return to the field, trail, course, road or court to enjoy sports again. In addition, I'll teach you how to increase your strength in a way that reinforces correct alignment with coordinated muscle mechanics. Finally, I'll present a new paradigm for sports training, an approach based on maintaining athletic durability for life. By the end, you'll be prepared to re-engage in sports with greater confidence, skill, and strength.

As we take this ride together, some of your preconceived ideas about healing, training, and sports may come into question. Stick with me when you start to doubt. My intention is to challenge your thinking about these issues. Recovering from chronic pain that has plagued you for some time is not a simple process. Something within you needs to change in order for you to heal. You are here and are reading this book for a different perspective; I am going to provide you with an alternative approach. Then you can choose what you do with the information.

Imagine understanding your pain instead of fearing it. Imagine having the tools not only to relieve it but also to prevent future injury. Envision being able to rely on yourself, not dependent on anyone else, for your healing. Picture regaining confidence in your body, knowing that you are balanced and strong in your structure. Imagine no longer feeling like your body is a ticking time bomb, just waiting for the next episode of pain and injury. Envision trusting your body to support you in all of your sports without having to baby your joints or worry about possible body failure. Realize that you are empowered to take action and make your pain go away for good. This book will show you how.

Ready—Set—Let's Go!

Throughout this book I will give you guidance, suggestions, and example exercises. However, this is not a step-by-step recipe approach to recovery. I do not believe in that model. Every client with knee pain should not be treated the same. Each client is unique. As you will read, my story and that of many of those I've helped would not fit into a generic stepwise progression to pain relief. Rather, my aim with this book is to give you information for consideration. What I present is not the common path to recovery. Instead of providing a recipe for you to follow, my goal is broader. I want to spark your curiosity and have you begin to question how injuries and pain are commonly treated. I hope to inspire you to investigate your thinking and the approach you have been following to heal. Ultimately, my quest is to expand your mindset and empower you to take purposeful action.

Winning the Injury Game is divided into three sections. Where you begin reading depends on where you are right now. The book is set up to take you from initial injury and pain back to athletics. So, if you are currently hurting, you're advised to start with the first section, "Align Your Mind," and work through the book sequentially. For those who want to dive right into the nuts and bolts of posture alignment, you'll want to start in the second section, "Align Your Body." If you are an athlete looking for guidance on training to prevent pain and injury, the third section, "Align Your Training," is where you'll want to begin.

In this book, I use many client stories along with my own. Some of these anecdotes are written in their words, and some in mine, with their critique. Many of the names are true, used with permission, while a fair portion have been changed to respect personal privacy. I've done my best to include perspectives from both genders, and I often switch between referring to "him" or "her" in my examples.

As you read my experiences, I urge you not to compare yourself too closely with me. We are all different and one-of-a-kind individuals. As I wrote this book, I realized there are very few joints I haven't had an issue with at some point along the way. This is not the norm for the clients I work with, and probably not for you, either. My path to recovery was long. The intention of this book is to make yours shorter.

This book includes "Game Winning Strategies" at the end of each chapter. I share my healing journey and those of my clients as examples in this book, but my ultimate goal is to help you along your path. These strategies will give you ways to maintain focus on your journey and to keep you involved in your process as you read. Many of the strategies involve reflective writing. I suggest you designate a separate notebook or journal with plenty of blank pages for these exercises. You could also use the computer, but I find the physical act of putting pen to paper more liberating. You won't be plagued by squiggly red lines when you misspell a word or have to concentrate on your typing. You'll be able to just let the words flow. I encourage you to write as much as you can in response to each inquiry. You might set a timer for each question, perhaps three to five minutes. You'll be surprised with what surfaces the longer you explore your thoughts on these topics. I know it is tempting to just flip right by these interactive sections of the book, but I do encourage you to at least read what's there and think about how you'd respond, even if you don't actually do the exercises. These are designed to help you gain a better understanding of yourself, which can aid your healing.

Book resources, including copies of the assessments, and videos of the exercises are located at www.thepfathlete.com/resources. I encourage you to take advantage of these free resources so you can repeat the assessments in the future and learn proper exercise form.

Have fun with the material and let me know what you think—good and bad. I spent years of my life writing this book, and I'd love to hear your feedback. Please make a comment or write a book review on the Pain Free Athlete Facebook page, www.facebook.com/painfreeathlete, or send me an email, jessica@thepfathlete.com, with your thoughts.

Happy Reading!

Align Your Mind

1

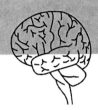

Healing is Possible!

*Y*our body is wonderfully resilient. It wants to serve you and make possible all the sports and activities you love. I know this is hard to hear right now; it might seem like your world has ended and a part of you died with your injury. But trust me: you can regain all you had and more. Your pain is only temporary. You *will* get better. I don't know how long it will take, but if you can be open to different possibilities and are willing to put in the effort required, you will recover.

You can do this! I've done it. Let me show you how.

My Story

All I wanted was to keep up with my husband while mountain biking. Many women have the same ambition. It seemed a reasonable goal. I neglected to consider that my husband, Ken, was a former professional mountain biker and extremely gifted in floating over technical terrain and bombing the downhills. On casual group rides, he regularly left everyone in his dust.

In my continued attempts to chase Ken down, my fitness greatly improved, leading me to become a professional mountain bike racer myself. I joined a professional women's team and traveled the country and the world on my bike. In 2004, I had the privilege of wearing the red, white and blue stars and stripes for Team USA at the *Marathon Mountain Bike World Championships* in Austria. I was at the peak of my athletic career—*or was I?*

Obviously, I could ride my bike fast and with skill, but is that the definition of wellness? If you looked beyond my pedaling prowess, the signs

13

of my fading health were evident. Two left knee surgeries, a torn quadricep muscle, recurring stomach upset, chronic sinus infections, repeating ankle pain, debilitating menstrual cramps, aching in my right shoulder and frequent bouts of severe neck tightness all led to fatigue and loss of motivation for cycling, training and living.

Fitness and Athletics ≠ Health and Wellness

I suffered repeated injuries and pain because I didn't have "athletic durability." According to the Postural Restoration Institute© (PRI), "Durability is a word meaning the ability to withstand wear, pressure, or damage. It is associated with an athlete's ability to have a relatively long continuous useful life without requiring an inordinate degree of maintenance."[1] This is my goal for you, to defeat your current injury and pain and increase your athletic durability during the process so you can enjoy sports long-term, without repeated breakdowns that require lots of maintenance. To perform at your highest level and achieve athletic durability, a balance between the 3 Domains of Performance—Biological, Fitness and Athletic—is required. Optimal performance is reached where these three domains intersect, as shown in Figure 1-1.

The Biological domain refers to how well all of your body systems—respiratory, vascular, circulatory, immune, musculoskeletal and so on—integrate together. This is the domain of your injury and pain. The Fitness domain refers to being in good physical shape. It is a measure of your cardiovascular endurance, strength, power, flexibility, etc. The Athletic domain refers to the specific movements and skills required for your sport. In the Athletic domain, the body is pushed beyond its normal boundaries through purposeful training to prepare for competition. A durable athlete can push the limits of his athletics while still respecting his biological performance. When I started having pain, I disregarded my biology in pursuit of greater athletic achievement. I could perform in the fitness and athletic performance domains, but I was falling apart in the biological domain. I didn't have athletic durability, which is why I only had one full season at top form as a professional mountain biker.

Our society idolizes athletes as visions of health, strength and ultimate fitness. Unfortunately, this is often not the case. Athletes are tenacious and determined individuals eager to push past points of pain and discomfort that

3 DOMAINS OF PERFORMANCE

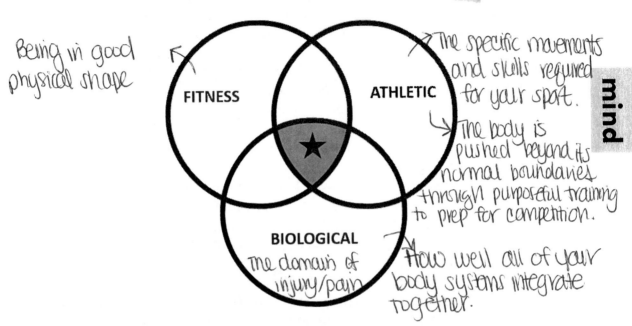

Being in good physical shape

FITNESS

ATHLETIC → The specific movements and skills required for your sport.

→ The body is pushed beyond its normal boundaries through purposeful training to prep for competition.

mind

BIOLOGICAL
The domain of injury/pain

How well all of your body systems integrate together.

Figure 1-1. The star in the intersect represents optimal performance.

Image used with permission from the Postural Restoration Institute® © 2016.
PRI Integration for Fitness and Movement Course Manual, www.posturalrestoration.com.

many people would not endure. We adhere to the philosophies of "mind over matter" and "no pain, no gain," willing to sacrifice our bodies to excel in our sport. We tolerate chronic pain—and inflict lasting injuries in our pursuit of success.

It doesn't *have* to be this way. But some people, like me, only learn the hard way. Despite my body's obvious signals of distress, I continued the abuse with more bike racing, ultra-marathon cross-country ski racing, and running—including sprint intervals—despite my doctor's warning after my first knee surgery never to run again. As long as I could still do these things, I rationalized that I was fine. *Big mistake!*

Of course, the stress of the workouts and competitions took its toll. It wasn't long before I damaged my left knee to the point of needing a third surgery. And I didn't stop there. Still dense to my body's messages, I pushed myself until pain in my left hip forced me to listen. Walking became a struggle as I limped from medical professional to complementary therapist, trying to find the easy answer and quick solution. I pursued several different "fixes": massage therapy; chiropractic adjustments; the use of heat, ice and anti-inflammatories; physical therapy; various forms of exercising; complete rest; Chinese herbs; acupuncture and yoga. None of these remedies relieved my symptoms for long. Although my MRI and X-rays didn't reveal anything conclusive, surgery seemed to be my only option.

After several months without relief, I underwent an exploratory arthroscopic surgery of my hip. Since recovery from my previous arthroscopic knee surgeries had been fast, and I was back on my bike within weeks, I expected the same after my hip procedure. And that's when everything changed. The hip operation hadn't been the "cure" to my problem. I soon discovered that it was merely the first step in what would be a long, challenging recovery. The torn hip labrum (cartilage) was repaired during the operation, but more significant was the diagnosis of severe (stage 4) hip osteoarthritis. As the doctor put it, I had a hole in my hip that was bone on bone. It would be years until I would comfortably mountain bike again.

My cycling quest took me from the highs of international competition to the lows of incessant pain and immobility. It was a difficult transition. My hard, narrow bike seat had been replaced with soft couch cushions. I couldn't exercise, which was my only outlet for the stress that was building. And not exercising was raising my anxiety to new heights as I felt my once exceptional fitness declining daily. I had lost a large segment of my social support circle since I wasn't out riding and competing. My eating habits had to change to compensate for my lack of movement and to control my escalating fear of gaining weight. Overall, I felt hopeless for my future. *What was life without sport?*

Fortunately, I had a dedicated massage therapist, Susan, who urged me to try the Egoscue Method®,[2] a pain relief approach through posture alignment. Although skeptical, I began reading *Pain Free*[3] by Pete Egoscue, an anatomical physiologist who founded the first Egoscue Method® Clinic in 1971. I experimented with the hip exercises outlined in the book and sought out guidance from an Egoscue® certified therapist. I'll expand on my experience with Egoscue® posture alignment therapy in Chapters 4, 6 and 8.

My path to healing was not quick, effortless or straightforward. In the beginning of my posture therapy, my pain increased. *Ouch!* It was my fault. I still had an athlete's mentality of "more is better," and when my body wasn't responding, I pushed even harder, increasing the intensity and repetitions of the restorative exercises. This only made things worse. My body couldn't do the basic movements correctly, so it compensated—cheating with other muscles and joints—to get the job done. By doing more, I increased the strain in the muscles that were already over working, thus escalating my pain. I had to re-learn how to move and stop powering through like I had always done. Sometimes, "less is more," and this was a very hard lesson for me to learn.

Despite increased pain and lack of progress, I continued with the Egoscue® posture alignment therapy. Intuitively, I knew that if I couldn't do these elementary movements, such as bringing my shoulder blades together, engaging my gluteal muscles evenly, and maintaining a static aligned posture without fatiguing, I had no chance of participating in more complex activities—cycling, hiking, skiing—without inflicting more stress and strain on my joints. I learned that it is the *position and condition* of the body brought into sports that matters most. Because I was out of balance when I played, I compensated and repeatedly suffered injuries.

A few months into my Egoscue® posture alignment therapy program, I began to feel more at ease in my body. My brain and muscles had learned to communicate, which led to greater strength and more efficient movement patterns. I could finally contract my left gluteal muscles—*hurrah!* With improved alignment and muscle coordination, I was able to pursue most sports again without pain, including once-forbidden activities like running.

Although I could do nearly everything I wanted to do, I still had pain when cross-country skate skiing. And the back pain I had at the beginning of my therapy had not abated completely. I also had intermittent problems with my feet, shoulders and neck. Considering how much I had gained, however, I felt this was okay and was willing to live with it, at least for a while. I knew deep down, though, that I hadn't reached the end of my healing journey. I knew that there was more work to be done. I just wasn't ready to face it yet, and I didn't know what to do next.

Five years later with my pains still lingering, I ended up in a course, Myokinematic Restoration, hosted by the Postural Restoration Institute® (PRI)[4] to fulfill CEUs (continuing education units). *Wow!* This course rocked my world. It was a totally new way of thinking about posture and a radically different approach to healing the body. I was instantly hooked, especially when I couldn't do the exercises. This just challenged me. Mind you, I was completely devastated, as I had already done so much work to recover. I asked myself, *When am I NOT going to be the most screwed up person in the class?*

Egoscue® and Postural Restoration® are both posture alignment techniques. They both have the same goal: returning symmetry to the skeleton. Both treat the body as a connected unit, with a focus on balancing the pelvis and strengthening the surrounding musculature. Both approaches strive to achieve correct body position before doing strengthening exercises. The Egoscue Method® uses exercises and stretches to realign the body, lengthening what is tight and strengthening what is weak. Postural Restoration® is also exercise-based and strongly integrates other systems of the body, primarily the respiratory and neurological systems. Attaining alignment of the axial skeleton—sacrum, spinal column, ribs, sternum and cranium—through efficient breathing mechanics and diaphragm positions is the essence of Postural Restoration®.[4] The position of all other soft tissues and joints in the body stems from this vital center. Breathing is also the regulating switch between the sympathetic, "fight-or-flight," and parasympathetic, "rest and digest," nervous systems. Being stuck in the sympathetic nervous system (SNS), as I was, leads to postural changes and the inability to initiate correct movement patterns. Postural Restoration® also acknowledges the inherent internal asymmetries within our bodies, which leads to overuse of some muscle groups while weakness develops in others.[1] (This will be explained further in Chapters 9-11.)

With the addition of Postural Restoration® to my regimen, I was finally able to conquer my back pain and skate ski pain-free. Although I had grown stronger with the Egoscue Method® exercises, I was still lacking in my core alignment, breathing mechanics and movement patterns. I was stuck in an overly dominant right-sided pattern, which was always firing up my right lower back muscles. Through Postural Restoration® training, I learned how to turn off the muscle patterns that were holding my core askew, restricting my breathing and keeping my back muscles tight.

Since my injuries, I have participated in the *American Birkebeiner* ski marathon, completed the *joBerg2c*—a 500-mile mountain bike race over nine days, run a trail marathon, raced a solo 12-hour mountain bike event, competed in *National Masters* Cross-Country Ski Races, lowered my golf handicap, participated in a 100-mile gravel cycling race, and continue to be on the starting line for many local and regional athletic competitions. In the beginning of my healing journey, I doubted I would ever be able to compete at a high level again, and I never imagined I'd feel strong enough to take on even harder challenges. I've now learned: Never say never.

Another profound benefit of my recovery is my enhanced mental and emotional outlook. No longer do I fear my body and feel as though it has abandoned me, slowly falling apart, joint by joint. I'm not waiting for the next catastrophe and surgery anymore. I have greater confidence in my body, knowing it is not fragile but is actually very tough, capable of supporting me in all of my athletic pursuits. With my heightened body-mind connection, I am aware of subtle changes—an unusually tight left hip muscle, slight but consistent pain in my right heel upon awakening in the morning, small losses in joint mobility or strength—and can take action before injuries occur.

To re-enter sports and competition, I had to change my philosophy about training. "No pain, no gain" is no longer my motto. I take a wholistic approach to my workouts, meaning that I condition not only my physical body, but also practice strategies to improve my mental and emotional performance. (Please note that throughout this book I used the word "wholistic," with a "w," to refer to a whole person approach to sports training; and "holistic," with an "h," to refer to a healing path that encompasses complementary and alternative methods.) I can now listen to and respect my body, integrate rest and recovery rituals, engage in a variety of activities, refine my sports technique and strengthen my body from the inside out with functional movements.

We athletes are designed to play sports throughout life. Injuries may happen along the way, but this does not mean an end to our days on the track, at the gym or in the water. As I have seen with myself and with my clients, the body has an incredible ability to regenerate and heal itself if you are willing to tune into its signs and take appropriate action. This may mean going back to the fundamentals of movement and postponing harder workouts or heavy weight-lifting for a while. But it is worth it. I feel fitter and healthier now than when I was overtraining as a professional athlete. By taking a holistic approach to my healing, I gained "athletic durability." I haven't had a major setback since starting down this path. *Give the body what it needs, and it will repay you with pain-free play for years to come!*

mind

Your Story

Now you've heard my story. What's yours? What story are you telling yourself about your injury and pain? In *The Power of Story*, Dr. Jim Loher, a world-renowned performance psychologist, explains that we are compelled to create stories to explain what happens to us: "Stories impose meaning on the chaos, they organize and give context to our sensory experiences which otherwise might seem like no more than a fairly colorless sequence of facts."[5]

Whether you are conscious of it or not, you have created a story around your injury and pain. To make sense of your experience, you have assigned significance to your current situation. The fact is, you hurt and cannot exercise like you want—period. There are many ways you can perceive this. As Loher explains, "Story is our creation of a reality... They [our stories] may or may not take us where we ultimately want to go."[5]

Upon suffering my hip injury, the story I told myself was one of being a victim to a body that had forsaken me. I told myself all kinds of negative things: I was weak. My body was flawed. My friends and competitors could train as much or more than I could without injury. There must be something wrong with me! I had cared for myself the best way I knew how and ended up sadly disappointed for my efforts. My thoughts were, *Why me? Why did this happen? Not another joint gone bad! It's not fair. I don't deserve this pain. Someone else must be to blame—my doctor? my coach? my training partners? Who?*

Does this sound familiar? Can you relate to the story I was telling myself? Do those same words go through your mind? I wouldn't be surprised, as I've heard these statements from my clients many times. We feel as though our body has betrayed us. The body that had supported us for so many years has failed, no longer letting us do what we want. And we are furious, scared, frustrated, resentful and heartbroken about it. We want someone else to fix it, NOW! We are willing to do anything to make the chronic pain go away. All we want is to be better so that we can continue on with our lives as before.

This negative thinking was not going to take me to where I ultimately wanted to go. Rather, it was going to keep me stuck in pain. Acting helpless leaves us with few options for healing. Everything is beyond our control when we're victims. In order to heal, you need to take an active, powerful role in your own healing process. Only then will you be successful.

Changing the Story

I had to change my story. I had to stop blaming others and my sports for my injury. (Mountain biking was *not* the cause of my pain.) I had to take responsibility for my health and stop looking to someone else to cure me, to terminate my eternal quest for the easy answer and quick fix. I needed to cease viewing myself as broken and unfixable. I had to dissociate from my diagnosis of severe osteoarthritis and stop identifying myself as a sufferer of an incurable, degenerative, lifelong disease that would inevitably lead to a hip replacement. I had to quit telling myself that I would not get better and back to athletics. I could not just accept that playing sports was to become a memory, a pleasure of the past not to be in my future. If I wanted to fully heal and return to competitive sports, it was essential that I stopped buying into these beliefs.

Making these changes wasn't easy for me. I want to make your journey from pain to activity smoother. Within the pages of this book, I will take you inside the process I went through to change my story. I will share with you how I altered my perceptions about my injury, changed my beliefs about healing, improved my mental outlook on chronic pain, balanced my body and consequently created a new reality—a reality full of hope for the future and a continuously expanding circle of activities, and a reality that has taken me exactly where I wanted to go.

Now it's your turn. Time to start your journey and take your first steps on your healing path toward your ultimate reality. We'll begin your holistic healing journey in the cognitive realm. You'll become aware of any blocks or resistance your mind is creating that may be counterproductive to your recovery. As you'll discover, your mind has a powerful impact—positive or negative—on your ability to heal. We'll start by addressing your thoughts and emotions about the most obvious aspect of your injury: your pain.

Summary

Healing is possible for you! The story you tell yourself about your injury and what you believe is possible impacts the truth of this statement. To return to sports and prevent future injuries, you'll need to re-build your Biological domain of performance, which is failing you now. Once this area is solid, you can safely increase the demands on your body with fitness and athletics. Recovering from chronic injury and pain may require exploring areas of your life you had not considered as contributing factors. Keeping an open mind, being persistent, and taking a holistic approach will bring you years of pain free activity, renewed body confidence, and ease of mind.

You can do this. Let's get started!

Game Winning Strategies

1. ### Prioritize Your Biological Performance

   Biological performance should be the pillar upon which fitness and athletics are supported and enabled.

   Fitness and Athletics ≠ Health and Wellness

   What health/wellness issues might you want to address?

   What is the first step you need to take?

   When are you going to take this action?

2. ### Know Your Story

   Become aware of your pain and injury story by writing it down. Look beneath the words to find the beliefs you hold about healing, your body, sports and more. If you don't like your story, start taking small steps toward change.

   What one thing can you do today to start moving in the direction of a better story—a story that you would be proud to tell?

mind

2

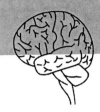

Reinterpreting Your Pain

*W*hat is pain? Here is my definition: Pain is a sensation that provides you with information about how your body is functioning. It cautions you that something is wrong.

In his book, *Painful Yarns*,[1] G. Lorimer Moseley, professor and leading clinical and research physiotherapist who specializes in the study of human pain at the University of South Australia, likens pain to the warning lights on a car dashboard. While hitchhiking in Australia, as he was taking a turn at the wheel for the weary driver who had picked him up, he noticed that one of the warning lights on the car dashboard became illuminated. Concerned, he questioned the car owner about the indicator light. The owner responded that it was nothing to worry about since it had been on before. Becoming increasingly nervous, as he knew from previous experience that ignoring a warning light can mean trouble, Moseley persisted that they stop to check the car. In response, the owner of the car reached up under the dashboard and pulled out the globe of the light. No more light, no more problem. As they continued driving, this happened twice more—for a total of three globes removed from the dashboard. When the fourth light came on, the car owner took a more drastic tactic and pulled the fuse so no lights appeared on the dash. Fortunately, they arrived safely at their destination. The next day, however, as the car owner was heading out of town, the steering and brakes went out, and the car caught fire and crashed. The driver survived with injuries.

The moral of the story: pain, like lights on a car dashboard, is a warning signal that things are not in harmony within your body. Failing to pay attention to these warnings can be very dangerous.

Ignoring My Pain

Pain can take on many forms, such as burning, tingling, numbness, stabbing, aching, or throbbing. It can also go undetected because your brain might not register the sensation as pain. Uneven muscle tightness, a nagging soreness, or a general feeling that something is not right is easily brushed off as just having a bad day or as being part of the price you pay to play. Since it's not registering as "painful," your mind doesn't warn you that it's potentially harmful. These are the small annoyances that can develop into severe pain and injury. Here is an example from my life when I ignored these subtle signals.

> When I started jogging again after my two knee surgeries, my left knee would complain softly and not feel quite right when I was done. It didn't hurt per se, but it didn't feel stable or unaffected by the pounding, either. Since the discomfort would diminish within a few hours, it was quickly forgotten until the next time I was out on the track. This cycle would repeat for weeks. The pain gradually intensified, and the recovery time lengthened. Because my knee did eventually "improve" and feel "better," I continued to run.
>
> In the beginning, the "funny" feeling would only happen after I ran. As the joint deteriorated, the discomfort was present from the first stride. Interestingly, my knee pain lessened the more I jogged. So, I rationalized that my knee was warming up, and if it improved as I ran, I couldn't be doing any permanent damage. Ha! Subsequent removal of 80% of frayed articular cartilage under my kneecap proved me wrong.

Body pain and mental desire are a dangerous combination. The one that wins is the one that talks the loudest. Initially, the excitement of jogging again overwhelmed the inconvenience of minor knee pain. With time, the voice of my knee rose from a faint whisper to a pleading, full-lung scream. In my mind, I desperately wanted to stay active, pursuing sports to the exclusion of the messages relayed from my body. Propelled by athletic aspirations, I ignored common sense, failed to respect my body, and continued pushing when I knew that stopping was the right thing to do. Another surgery was my reward for being deaf to my body's pain warning signals.

Catastrophic injuries happen because we do not listen to our bodies. If I had heeded my pain early and had corrected my postural imbalances and dysfunctional movement patterns, I might have avoided a third knee operation. However, I refused to appreciate my pain and continued to literally run through it—and from it. My body could not heal, could not recover, and instead it grew weaker and more damaged. The only way the body can regenerate is by reducing the internal stress, which is what the pain was acknowledging. I overrode this protective body signal and ultimately paid the price.

Athletics Teaches Us to Override Pain

Let's be honest. If, as athletes, we always listened when our bodies complained and begged for rest, we wouldn't get very fit or win many races. Training for sports is hard and painful. Pushing yourself through that tenth sprint interval when your quads are burning and lungs are straining *hurts. A lot!* Your body sends all kinds of messages that it doesn't want to endure this agony anymore and pleads for you to stop. But, you know that to gain greater fitness and to have a chance of being on the podium next time, you must keep going.

This is what I call "good pain." It is the type of pain that will make you stronger and faster. It is a necessary part of structured athletic training. The problem is, to experience this "good pain" and achieve the training benefits it provides, you must override the discomfort in your body. You must talk yourself into voluntarily inflicting pain on yourself. Have you ever heard an athlete describe her race experience as a "sufferfest?" Heck, there are races with that name, and others enticing participants with an equally miserable experience—"*Pajarito Punishment*," "*Galena Grinder*," "*La Tierra Torture*"—just to name a few events I have done. We athletes are an interesting breed. We seek out the pain. The harder and more anguish involved, the better.

A problem arises, however, when you do not differentiate between "good" and "bad" pain. Injuries happen and become severe when you fail to recognize and take action when you feel the "bad pain." This is the pain that is not the result of physical exertion: it is the result of tissue or joint damage. By being in the habit of suppressing your body's voice, which includes pain, you often miss this news flash. Or, you hear it, and like me, choose to ignore it, hoping it will just go away on its own.

Changing Your Relationship With Pain

Why do we work so hard to avoid the "bad pain?" Quite simply, because it makes us afraid. We fear what we do not understand. We easily comprehend the hurt of hard training, but we do not know how to interpret pain coming from our back, knees, or shoulders. For many of us, the human body is an enigma. We do not know how to assess our body pain, so we immediately associate it with something very bad. Since we are scared and often do not know what to do about the pain, we tend to jump to irrational conclusions: we assume it must signal that something is terribly wrong, and we fear that it will require invasive procedures such as surgery or injections to correct. We believe that since pain keeps us from playing, it is to be avoided at all costs.

I'd like to challenge you to open up to the possibility of considering pain differently. What if, instead of being an indicator of impending doom and forced inactivity, you could come to appreciate your pain? What if you could come to realize that pain has a positive side? What if you could come to understand that pain helps to keep you safe and healthy?

Pain has a dual role in your body: communication and protection. It is the body's last resort mechanism to get your attention. You have ignored the subtle signals that your body has sent you: the strange feelings, muscle tightness, reduced range of motion, and so on. To make you take notice and stop your destructive behavior, your body is forced to take harsh action and makes you hurt—terribly. Your pain is trying to help you prevent further or more serious injury. *That is a good thing!*

Connecting With Your Pain

Do you hear what your body is saying to you? More importantly, do you listen? As you have read, like many athletes, I didn't want to hear from my body when it provided messages that were counter to what my mind wanted. I blocked and rationalized my physical signals of soreness, pain and fatigue. When my body had good things to say, I didn't listen, either; feeling good was expected.

How connected are you with your body? Are you like I was, teaching yourself to disregard your body's innate intelligence? Right now, pain is the information your body is providing, loud and clear. Many of us do not like or want this negative news, so we might choose to dissociate from it. This is a natural response to pain. We want to deny it, escape from it, forget about it, and hope that it just disappears. So, we may take an aspirin or ibuprofen to numb the feeling. Unfortunately, in many cases, the pain does not dissipate for long. It stays with us, urging us to acknowledge it and take appropriate action. However, ignoring the pain and continuing to abuse and condemn our body for the pain will only make the injury worse and prolong healing.

Instead of fearing and fleeing the pain, Jon Kabat-Zinn, Ph.D., founder of the Stress Reduction Clinic at the University of Massachusetts Medical Center, advises going into the pain and fully experiencing it to overcome it. His Mindfulness-Based Stress Reduction (MBSR) program combines mindfulness meditation, body awareness, and yoga for healing.[2] These strategies are all focused on deepening your relationship and connection with your body. According to Gary Schwartz, Ph.D., a psychologist known for his work in energy healing at the University of Arizona (my alma mater—Bear Down Wildcats!), connection is essential for good health. Schwartz proposes that disconnection is largely caused by disattention.[2] We do not pay attention to our body's signals, we do not listen to our pain, and our body systems get out of balance. In his model of connectedness and health, it all flows downstream from disattention.

Disattention ➡ Disconnection ➡ Disregulation ➡ Disorder ➡ Disease

Fortunately, you can reverse this pattern and get back to health by becoming connected with yourself and your body, starting with attention.

Attention ➡ Connection ➡ Regulation ➡ Order ➡ Ease/Health

So, to rid yourself of the pain, you must pay attention to your body, listen to it, and become connected with it—physically, mentally, emotionally, and spiritually.

Kabat-Zinn encourages his mindfulness meditation students to face their pain and be with it moment by moment. When they can stay with their pain in the present moment, they often find they can continue to be with it for longer and longer durations. If you're like me, getting closer to your pain sounds like the last thing you want to do. After all, who wants to snuggle up with what is causing them so much misery? It goes back to our fear of the unknown. Just like most of us do not want to enter a dark, cold cave because we don't know what might be lurking beyond, we do not want to delve into our pain, unsure of what we might uncover. We're afraid of finding out that the pain is worse than anticipated. We prefer to live in safe ignorance.

Knowing Your Pain

When you go into your pain, you may realize that not all pain is the same. I've previously discussed "good" and "bad" pain, the first being a normal part of sports training, and the latter, a pain indicating potential damage to your body. If colors were applied to these, I would make "good" pain white and "bad" pain black, as shown in Figure 2-1.

Figure 2-1. A large gray area exists between the two ends of the pain spectrum.

The gray areas within your pain are often hidden from your perception. For many, when it comes to pain, it is black or white. Either you have pain, or you don't have pain. Learning to differentiate between the shades of gray within your pain, the subtle changes in the severity, frequency and duration of your pain, can be an important part of your recovery process, providing motivation and encouragement. However, if you cannot acknowledge and appreciate your movement within the gray area on the pain spectrum from black toward white, then you may remain stuck in pain. This was the case for my client, Lynn.

When Lynn initially came to me for posture therapy, she was frustrated and defeated by the pain throughout her body. Prior to seeing me, Lynn had sought out many experts and tried numerous body-focused therapies to heal her pain, including various forms of hands-on bodywork, stretching regimens, strengthening programs, and many different custom foot orthotics and shoes; unfortunately, she was not improving. At the start of each session, I would ask Lynn how she was doing. In response, she would list her numerous ailments from head to toe, commenting that she hurt nearly everywhere. It would be the same each time I saw her. I would ask how she did with her exercises, if she noticed any changes in her body, and how her sports were going, in the hopes of finding an area in which she had success. She rarely had anything positive to report. She would not admit even the slightest improvement in her condition.

When Lynn was a young runner, she had an eating disorder. Unhappy with her physical appearance, she protected herself by dissociating from her body. She shut down all communication from her body, choosing to disregard the information it was trying to send. This had a lasting effect, which made it nearly impossible for her to differentiate sensations in her body. All she could feel was pain, and she always perceived it as being the same.

After several months of working together with no improvement, I asked Lynn, "Why do you keep coming back? Why do you keep doing the posture exercises if they aren't helping?" It didn't make any sense to me, and I was determined to either shock her into a change or release her as a client. Fortunately, my risky question worked, as Lynn explained:

That made me stop and think. Perhaps there was some improvement, but I never dared to acknowledge it, lest it slip away like always before, leaving me with yet another layer of disappointment and discouragement. Instead I chose to just keep grunting through the day, doing whatever I could and hoping that someday, magically, I would wake up and not be in pain. Like many other things in my life, and in the tradition of true perfectionism, everything was black and white. There was no gray. That day with Jessica, where I realized what I was doing, was one of those pivotal sessions that was life changing. What if I questioned my beliefs and looked deeper? What if I really started living inside of my body again and paid attention to subtle changes and shifts? What if I accepted and acknowledged where I was, rather than where I wanted to be? What if I could celebrate the small steps on my way to the ultimate goal of healing?

Recovery has become an interesting experiment for Lynn. She no longer denies her pain. Rather, she realizes that it is a source of information upon which her choices are made. Instead of choosing self-defeating thoughts, she now consistently opts for smarter choices that support her healing. Being able to feel more than pain, she can differentiate many sensations in her body. She recognizes when her muscles are lengthening, engaging and moving in synchrony and balance.

By experiencing the gray areas of her pain, Lynn now appreciates the steps she has made, giving her hope for healing. Without this free communication with herself, she felt hopeless. She wasn't able to notice her progress toward her ultimate goal of becoming pain free. Now, more conscious and able to openly acknowledge the changes in her body, Lynn can assess the effectiveness of her treatment. Adopting an attitude of curiosity, she can communicate with her body about what is shifting, what is working, and what needs to be modified to aid her recovery. With her enhanced body awareness, she can notice that her pains are dynamic, not a constant burden, and she has realized for the first time that some of her pain has disappeared. The way Lynn was viewing her pain was impeding her healing. She couldn't acknowledge even small, positive changes. Once she realized that pain exists on a spectrum and includes many shades of gray, Lynn was free to perceive her body and situation differently, which aided her recovery.

Pain Awareness Aids Healing

Awareness is one of the first steps toward becoming pain free. You cannot change what you are not aware of, and if you do not change, you will not heal. Connecting with your pain and being able to characterize it accurately accelerates your recovery. Pain is subjective and hard to assess from the outside. Coaches, like me, are at a disadvantage when working with chronic pain clients. I cannot feel what you feel; I can only rely on you for detailed descriptions of your sensations.

Becoming aware of the subtleties and gradations in your pain may be a new experience for you. To guide you in developing your pain awareness, here are a few sample questions: Is there anything that relieves your pain even slightly? Is there any position that makes your body feel more comfortable? That could be a big clue as to what is wrong. What movements exacerbate your pain? Does it hurt when you do X, but not Y? Is your pain constant, or do you notice it goes away at times? How would you describe your pain? When is the pain most severe? The more you know and can skillfully relate to your health care providers, the better they can serve you.

Since you may not comprehend the complexities of the body, you might feel intimidated and powerless; you might not believe you are qualified to assess your pain. This is understandable. However, *you are* the only one who can access your pain. I always tell my clients that we are working together as partners in their healing. I have external intelligence about their bodies, but they have the very powerful inside angle on what is going on. Sharing a role in your treatment is empowering and essential. Just as you often cannot heal yourself entirely alone, a practitioner cannot help without your input, and the better the information you provide, the more effective your treatment will be.

Your Brain Interprets Your Pain

Clinical Neurosciences Professor Dr. Lorimer Moseley says, "Pain is a construct of the brain."[3] Now to be clear, I am not suggesting that the pain is all in your head or that you are making it up. However, I do understand that can happen. During my healing, a therapist implied this was what was holding me back in my recovery process. He suggested I read anything by Dr. John E. Sarno, a physician and pioneer in the field of mind-body medicine. I did find this helpful. If you are interested in learning more, I'd recommend starting with his *New York Times* bestseller, *Healing Back Pain.*[4]

Back to Moseley's point: our soft tissues, by themselves, are unable to create the sensation of pain. It is not until the information about the damage reaches the brain that a determination is made about how to react. The brain interprets the situation and makes a judgment about the severity of the injury and the best way to respond. Depending on the circumstances and your previous experience with similar pain, the brain can choose to make the pain intense or barely noticeable.

mind

In his TED (2011)[3] talk and book, *Painful Yarns,*[1] Moseley tells his popular story of being bitten by an eastern brown snake, one of the deadliest snakes in the world. I highly recommend watching his presentation as he is quite entertaining. In his talk, he describes walking in the Australian bush, something he had done many times before, and feeling discomfort on the outside of his calf, a sensation that usually meant he was scratched by a twig. On this particular day, however, it was a snake bite. What is interesting to notice in his story is how his brain responds to the snake bite—along with his reaction the next time he is out walking after he'd been bitten.

As he explains it, he was walking along in the bush and felt a sensation on the outside of his calf. Upon sensing this, his brain surveyed the situation and surmised that it was not dangerous, so he continued walking with little pain. His brain had determined that he had been in the area before, had felt the same feeling on the same area of his body during the same phase of the gait (walking) cycle, and so it was not a threat—a notable injury to the body. It was merely a scratch by a twig. The reality was, he had been bitten by the often-deadly eastern brown snake and was lucky to have survived. Hence, when he was walking in the bush the next time and felt the same sensation on his leg, his brain sounded the alarm bells and made his leg hurt so much that he could not continue walking. His brain had the memory of almost dying the last time this had happened and was not going to let him ignore this "very serious threat." However, this time the injury turned out to be the familiar small scratch by a twig. Moseley's recent experience of being bitten by a snake influenced how his brain reacted to the pain. It was not the body injury itself, the scratch or snake bite on his leg, that dictated his behavior, but rather the brain's interpretation of the situation.

In his book *Explain Pain,* Moseley states that "the amount of pain you experience does not necessarily relate to the amount of tissue damage you have sustained,"[5] as his snake bite story demonstrates. Interestingly, back pain research has found that the amount of damage and pain experienced do not always correlate. A study by Jensen, et al., found people with no back pain had disc bulges and protrusions on their magnetic resonance imaging (MRI) scans.[6] Although damage was seen in the lumbar spines of these subjects, they did not feel any pain. Consequently, according to Moseley, this would mean that the brain did not perceive these body changes as a threat and did not register them as pain. How much you hurt, then, is influenced by other factors outside the amount of physical harm.

Pain is only one option the brain has as a response to a bodily injury. Moseley tells stories of people who don't feel pain even though their body has sustained a great trauma—soldiers who have been shot and surfers who have had their legs bitten off.[5] Due to the dangerous environment the people in these examples are in—war zones with enemy fire or the ocean waters—it is not in the brain's best interest to send the response of severe pain and immobilize the person. In that moment, the brain is more concerned with keeping the person safe and out of harm's way. Pain would jeopardize the victim's ability to flee the scene and get to safety.

The Meaning Behind Your Pain

Physical injury imposes movement limitations, but it might also signify a deeper personal loss. Often, it is what the pain and injury represent that causes the true suffering. For example, as Kabat-Zinn's meditation students stayed with their pain longer, they discovered it was not the negative bodily sensation itself that was the problem, but rather the way that they were thinking about and interpreting the pain in their minds.[2] During meditation, one of Kabat-Zinn's male students realized that it was not the unpleasant sensation in his back that was causing him the most pain. Rather, his greater suffering stemmed from not being able to work, an effect of his pain. As a result of his back injury, he had lost his income earning potential and the ability to provide for his family. Failing to fulfill this important role was a larger personal loss. This hurt more deeply than his back.[2]

In a 1999 study by Bianco, Malo and Orlick, athletes of the Canadian Alpine Ski Team who had sustained a serious injury or illness were interviewed. They found athletes suffered more depending on the timing and consequences of the injury. One of the interviewed athletes states, "I trained very hard for 3 years and the year I could qualify for the Olympics, I fell ill. It was a huge shock. I wanted to quit. It was morally and psychologically very difficult."[7] Additionally, an athlete who suffered a career-ending injury, one that caused him to never reach his goals, experienced heightened levels of loss and depression over an athlete who would recover to ski competitively again.[7]

Again, it is what the pain and injury represent that causes the true suffering. For the skiers the pain represented a lost opportunity to be in the Olympics, a chance that may never come again, and the realization of the end of a sports career. The important thing to take note of here is that the physical pain you feel can take on many meanings in your mind: I am getting older, I am not as fit as I was, I do not recover well, I am going to miss an important event, I am weak, I am not going to be able to be with my friends, and so on. These thoughts and the emotions they trigger are frequently what is really upsetting you about your injury. Luckily, your responses are within your control and can be changed. This can be seen in the example of my client, Sandra, who nearly gave up her dreams because of her pain. Here's her story, in her words:

> When I was 12 years old, I was diagnosed with scoliosis. I was told it was an irreversible condition. The doctor advised me to strengthen my back, and surgery was not likely to relieve the pain. At the time, I aspired to backpack the Grand Canyon with my friends and to carry my school backpack without pain. My dreams were out of reach. My pain reinforced that I was not good enough, no matter how hard I tried. For a pre-teen struggling with perfectionism, it was a hard thing to bear.
>
> I took up rock climbing to strengthen my back, but the pain kept me from feeling truly strong and capable. I stopped dreaming. Not yet 20, I felt as though my best athletic years were already behind me, and my body was going to slowly deteriorate.
>
> At 23, a chiropractor X-rayed my back and showed me that my spinal curvature was not caused by the shape of my vertebrae, but likely by soft tissue imbalances. This gave me the hope I needed to embark on a journey and pursue what I knew deep inside: I may be in pain and "broken" now, but I can heal. I desperately wanted to dream again.
>
> Recently, an orthopedic surgeon could not detect my scoliosis with palpation of my spine. Just over 20 years after my diagnosis the once obvious lateral curves are gone. I can say that I had scoliosis. I met my goal. I did it!
>
> In the process, I established a new relationship with my pain. I now see pain as a language. It may still be telling me about a physical problem; however, it may have more to say. It could be telling me

that I am stressed or not taking care of myself. When I find myself frustrated or fearful, I can notice and guide myself out of judgment and into self-care. By reaching for my dream, I did not just address my pain, but I changed. I grew taller (or at least straighter), stronger, and kinder to myself. It is a time to celebrate, to confidently believe in myself, and to dream again.

mind

Pain Associations

The brain draws conclusions between stimulus and pain.

When I was finally able to get back on my bike, over a year after my debilitating hip injury, I did so with reservations. For me, the bike had become a symbol of my pain. My mind had created a link between cycling and back pain. I expected to hurt when I rode, and for a long time I did. In my brain, bike = pain. In order to heal, I had to create new associations with my bike: bike = fun, bike = freedom, bike = friends.

Although the tissues in my back were no longer acutely damaged—most tissue damage heals in three to six months[8]—my brain was still creating pain in response to the "bike" stimulus. I was trapped in an old response pattern, which made biking, once my passion, into a misery. I had to retrain my response to the bike. Using deep, focused breathing and imagining my back muscles lengthening while I rode, I was able to keep my back muscles relaxed so that I wouldn't feel the familiar tightening as I pedaled.

On top of my physical discomfort on the bike, I also had mental and emotional ties to cycling. Prior to my injury, I had been a professional mountain biker. Shortly before my hip surgery, I competed in the International Mountain Bike World Cup race. This additional pressure of not being at the top of my form, as well as worrying about others viewing me as being slow and weak, only fed my pain experience on the bike. With time, and with the support and encouragement from others, I was able to let go of this self-image and enjoy riding again.

As a final example, one of my clients developed an association between his foot pain and closed-toe shoes. His feet were fine if he wore flip flops or sandals or if he went barefoot, but his feet would quickly hurt when he put on any pair of closed-toe shoes, regardless of fit. In order for him to heal, I had to make him aware of the association he had made between his foot pain and his shoes. Once he realized this, he was able to comfortably wear most of his shoes again.

Mind Awareness Aids Healing

Although you may not be familiar with the term "mind awareness," you are probably familiar with the concept of "body awareness." When I hear the term "body awareness," I associate this with becoming conscious of only my physical being. People who are body aware might consciously think things like, Is my muscle tight? Are my legs straight or bent? Is my weight balanced evenly on both feet when I stand? Are my shoulders level? "Body awareness" is very important to healing and is covered in more detail in Chapter 11.

To heal, a person needs two things: awareness of what is happening in the body and awareness of what is going on in the mind. Many times, a person's greatest pain is generated in the mind. Having the ability to get in touch with your mental, emotional and spiritual states can free you from some of this cognitive pain.

Questions to consider: Do you know what your inner voice is saying? Can you identify the emotions you are experiencing? Are you aware of how your injury is affecting your attitude, relationships and life purpose?

As an example, my husband Ken and I are both very active and find joy in getting outside and doing things together. When I was hurt, I often found myself jealous and depressed when he would go out and play sports without me. My injury created tension and stress within our relationship.

Although you cannot change your partner's desire to be active, acknowledging your response and communicating openly with your significant other can help. My client Helen provides another example of the effects an injury can have on one's emotions, meaning, and relationships.

> Helen deeply values family, and when I met her, she had a strong desire to be a mom. In her early thirties, she was ready to start having children when she endured a back injury. (More on Helen's back pain story in Chapter 5.) In addition to her physical pain, she suffered because of the disappointment she felt about waiting to have children. Her stress was also elevated by the realization that her time to start a family was dwindling, knowing that the risks of pregnancy increase with age. The consequences of Helen's injury went beyond herself and influenced her relationships with her husband and family, who were also looking forward to the possibility of children, grandchildren, and nieces and nephews.

mind

You know that you are in pain, but are you aware of what is going on in your psyche as a response? Becoming aware of what is going on in your head can help you make sense of your actions, especially when they are contrary to your goals. Realize that your injury is having far-reaching effects, and let yourself get in touch with the cognitive side of your pain. This is not weakness; it is empowerment. The next chapter delves into the typical mental and emotional response that come with being injured and gives several coping tools.

Summary

Pain often provokes fear when you hurt. You might be most afraid of not being able to continue playing. And, you may be apprehensive that the pain will negatively affect your physical lifestyle. Please keep in mind that pain has a positive side and acts as the body's communication channel and warning system. Sensing pain may actually prevent a more serious injury. In most cases, pain is trying to protect you.

Through sports you may have learned to ignore or override your pain. You may have developed a habit of downplaying and rationalizing your discomfort so the game could go on. To heal, you'll need to step into your pain and become familiar with it and how it changes. Pain is not black or white. It has many shades of gray. You'll want to stay alert for even small improvements in your pain as signs that you are getting better. Learn to embrace rather than flee from your pain to aid your recovery.

It is critical that you are aware of the pain in your body and mind. Ultimately, the brain decides how you respond to physical pain, and many of these responses—mental, emotional, and spiritual—are within your control and can be improved. Pain has widespread effects throughout your life. This cognitive suffering is often what hurts the most—particularly, the meaning you have attributed to your pain and injury.

Unknowingly, you may have developed associations between your pain and certain activities, movements, and sports. Disconnect these links to unlock your healing and return to activity.

> **Game Winning Strategies**

1. Define Pain

How you think about your pain can impact your ability to heal. Take a few minutes to answer the following questions.

What is your definition of pain?

What emotions do you connect with pain?

Reflecting on your answers above, how might your descriptions of pain be affecting your current situation?

2. Interpret Your Pain

Pain has several shades of gray. The intensity of the pain you feel is often times not solely correlated with the amount of body damage. Pain can influence multiple aspects of your life. Questions to consider:

What changes have you noticed in your pain?

How would you explain your observations to your healthcare provider?

What meaning have you attached to your pain? What does your pain represent?

What, if any, associations have you made with your pain?

What impact is your pain having on your relationships, outlook, and life purpose?

mind

3

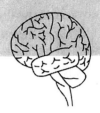

How Your Mind Responds to Injury

*I*f you're like me, it's normal to be experiencing a variety of strong emotions right now while you're hurting. Your emotional state is probably like a roller coaster. One minute you're happy and coping well, and the next, you're in tears and yelling at the dog for no reason. Please be reassured that whatever you are feeling right now is okay; it's a natural part of the healing process.

You have suffered a personal loss with your injury. A common response to such a trauma, as I will explain, is to grieve. Just like a dying patient, some injured athletes go through a grief cycle. Dr. Elisabeth Kübler-Ross, a Swiss-American psychiatrist, pioneered the five stages of grief while working with the terminally ill. She first published her famous book, *On Death and Dying,* in 1969. Through her interactions with the dying, she recognized a recurring emotional rhythm in her patients. She observed her patients initially expressing "denial and isolation," then "anger," followed by "bargaining," "depression," and finally "acceptance."[1] These are the five stages of the grief cycle, which will be discussed in this chapter.

The many emotions you are sensing right now reflect your stage of grief. Although people may progress through the stages sequentially, as outlined above, this is often not the case. A study by Brewer failed to find evidence that athletes move through these stages in an orderly fashion.[2] It has been suggested that an injured athlete typically does not go through these stages sequentially; instead, the athlete goes through more of a cyclical process. Other models, one of the most popular being *The Affective Cycle of Injury,* have been created to take into account this cyclical nature of athletic injury.[3] Since there doesn't seem to be consensus on an athlete's cognitive path through injury, I am going to use Dr. Kübler-Ross' model,[1] which has withstood the test of time, as the framework for my discussion. However, I do appreciate that athletes cycle through these stages, and that mental and

43

emotional healing, just like physical healing, is an individual process that follows different paths for each person. Regardless of the model used, it can be reassuring for you, the injured athlete, to understand that the grief and strong emotions you are feeling are ordinary responses to being injured.

The First Stage of Grief: Denial and Isolation

There's nothing wrong with me! When first injured, you may want to deny that there is a problem, so you continue to exercise through the pain, hoping it will spontaneously go away. Athletes have a great capacity for rationalization. They will use skewed logic to continue to do what they want to do, despite clear evidence from their body to the contrary. This was the case for my client, Gretchen.

Gretchen is a talented cyclist. She loves the feeling of being on two wheels. She is drawn to ride her bike; it helps her stay mentally balanced and happy. Upon suffering Achilles tendonitis, Gretchen kept riding. Even after doing a steep hike, which flared up her injury, she mounted her bike the next day. She was compelled to ride, and the pain wasn't that bad, so why not? As she pedaled, she could feel some discomfort, but she reasoned that it wasn't getting worse and would be okay. The doctor then told her to back off, so she took the recommended six weeks off. She thought that should be long enough for the injury to heal, and so, after six weeks, she eagerly resumed her cycling training. As happens to many of us, Gretchen could not outride her pain. During a road bike ride, Gretchen's husband saw her climbing up a steep hill, contorting her body to avoid the hurt. She felt the pain but kept trying to ride. After a few more miles, and after consulting with her husband, who verified her unbalanced pedaling and awkward body mechanics, she reluctantly stopped and got a ride home. It was obvious she was suffering and was pushing her body beyond its capabilities as she tried to deny her injury.

Gretchen was fortunate to have someone observe her destructive behavior and to help her realize the consequences of her actions. Many of us, without an outside perspective and left to our own devices, won't stop, even when our body begs for rest.

Gretchen's story leads into the second emotion that is associated with the first stage of grief: isolation. She mostly remembers the loneliness she felt upon realizing she would be sitting out almost all activity, even walking and hiking, for six whole weeks as it got warmer and warmer and nicer and nicer outside. It was springtime! She watched others riding. She imagined her cohort of training partners getting stronger every day. She felt left out, frustrated, and in her words, "quite pathetic."

You can be separated from your social group when you are not able to play, especially if you are frequently confined to your home. I recall feeling similar to Gretchen when I had my hip surgery during the summer of 2007. This is what I wrote in my journal:

> *Lying on the couch with fresh stitches in my thigh, the ice pack begins to drip, and my head is spinning from the pain medication. The sun is shining. I can see the mountains from my window. I yearn to be out on those trails but haven't ridden my bike for four months. Last summer, I was training for the Leadville 100 mountain bike race. This year, I'm stuck inside, watching the other cyclists ride by, leaving me behind.*

The isolation and hurt that athletes feel is physical, emotional, and social. I was physically separated from my cycling friends. They were exploring the outdoors, while I was home alone with my pain. Emotionally, I was segregated, feeling like nobody could relate to my plight. I desperately wanted someone to talk to, but I couldn't find many understanding ears. Socially, I elected to withdraw from my athletic circle. I couldn't bear to hang out with other athletes who were talking about their great adventures. I didn't want to attend local athletic events; it was just too hard to be on the sidelines.

Losing Your Identity

Mountain biking was what I did and how I defined myself. I was a professional mountain biker! When I wasn't able to ride my bike, I felt not only externally isolated but also internally disconnected.

Do you question who you are without sport? You have always identified yourself as an athlete, labeling yourself as a hiker, swimmer, rower, dancer, etc. If you have lost your ability to participate, you can no longer define your uniqueness through sport. How do you feel when you win a race or meet a challenging athletic goal? You feel good, right? As you should. You worked hard and were successful. Time for celebration! And as a result of accomplishing this athletic goal, you feel significant. According to life coach and motivational speaker Tony Robbins, one of our basic human emotional needs is significance. Robbins explains, "Some individuals will pursue this need [for significance] by competing with others."[4] So, sports can help us feel important and special. Did you know that you may be using sports participation as a way of meeting your need for significance? I had never thought of it this way, which is not surprising, since our authentic needs and deeper motivations reside on a subconscious level of awareness. Interestingly, these needs influence our emotions and drive our actions.[4]

Maybe that is why some athletes continue to exercise despite their pain. They do not have another way of meeting their need for significance. You probably know these people, as I do: the athlete who can barely limp to the chair lift but continues to ski down the mountain; the athlete who cannot drive for an hour comfortably in the car but rides a road bike century; the athlete who cannot walk without pain but insists on running long trail miles.

Robbins points out that the desire to meet our emotional needs can be either empowering or destructive.[4] On the negative side, people may go against their morals, values and beliefs (spiritual misalignment) to gain their needs. Perhaps the injured athlete knows that he should quit and is causing bodily harm with his actions. He values his body and wants to treat it with respect, but his need for significance is so strong that he literally cannot stop himself from participating in sport—regardless of the consequences.

In addition to significance, an injured athlete may continue to play when motivated by her needs for love and belonging, self-esteem, or self-actualization, as outlined in the top three tiers of Abraham Maslow's pyramid-shaped hierarchy of needs model,[5] as shown in Figure 3-1.

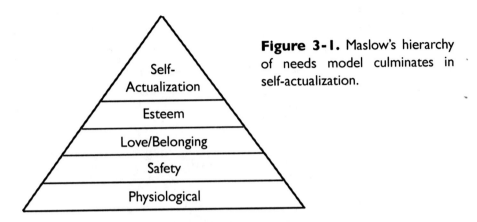

Figure 3-1. Maslow's hierarchy of needs model culminates in self-actualization.

mind

Maslow was a U.S. psychologist who changed the direction of psychology at his time by focusing on the positive aspects of human potential. He was a founder of Humanistic Psychology, with the ultimate goal of helping people reach self-actualization, which is at the top of his enduring hierarchy of needs model.[6] In his model, self-esteem and love and belonging are situated below self-actualization. Each level of the pyramid builds on the next. Self-actualization, or reaching one's potential, can only be achieved when all of the underlying needs are met and mastered. The top two tiers—self-actualization and self-esteem—are similar to Robbins' idea of significance in that they give a person self-worth; however, Maslow's idea of love and belonging could be met through participation on a sports team or by pleasing family or friends.

While in gymnastics, I knew girls who didn't care anything about the sport but who participated to gain affection from their parents. And, we have all seen the game on TV where the player hobbles off the field with what seems like a serious injury, only to return to the action a few minutes later, desperate to be part of the team. We've also watched the player on the sideline begging the coach to let him play, despite his pain and disability.

I see this in my friend Michael, who competes in many sports. He does not really enjoy the stress of racing, but he feels obligated to participate. As he says, "It's what's expected" by his team, his friends and himself. If he does not compete, he feels as though he is letting others down. It is the peer pressure, the need to be part of something, and the desire to be accepted into the group that pushes him to continue.

Another friend, Ashley, needs to validate her self-worth regularly by competing nearly every weekend. She needs to prove her superiority as an athlete to feel good about herself. The desire to retain your identity as an athlete is powerful, often serving to meet unknown psychological needs. This dependency on being seen as an athlete is especially strong if your life is not balanced, as you will read next.

You Are More Than an Athlete

Being an "athlete" is only one identity that defines you. There are many other roles you fulfill in life. In her book, *Feel the Fear . . . and Do It Anyway,* Susan Jeffers, Ph.D., psychologist and renowned author of 18 self-help books, discusses how people become needy and desperate when they lose things to which they are emotionally tied.[7] They feel as though they have little control over their circumstances. This can create great anxiety and fear.[7]

Daughter/Son	Friend	Parent/Grandparent
Employee/Employer	Brother/Sister	Relative
Spouse/Partner	**Athlete**	Community Member
Citizen	Pet Owner	Volunteer
Home Owner/Renter	Cause Activist	Traveler
Student	Teacher/Mentor	Hobbyist (Cook, etc.)

As an athlete, you may place a higher priority and feel a deeper responsibility to your sport than to other aspects of your life. You may even neglect your other roles and focus more on the sport—so when you're injured and can no longer play the sport, it seems disastrous. Dr. Jeffers uses the "Whole Life Grid"[7] to demonstrate life balance. The grid has nine boxes filled with the different components of life, such as family, leisure, and work, among others. I have adapted and expanded this grid structure to illustrate some of the different roles you may perform in your life. Your grid may have different roles, of course. The completed grid is an example.

If your grid is full, losing your identity as an athlete will be less traumatic. However, if your grid is narrowly focused like the one below, then losing your identity as an athlete can be devastating.

```
┌─────────────────────────┐
│         Athlete         │
└─────────────────────────┘
```

Of course, you have other roles in life, but if you are not as dedicated to them, or if you put little importance on them, the loss of this essential role of being an athlete will be catastrophic. Your view of life may have become distorted due to your emotional investment in and your attachment to sports. In this scenario, when you cannot play, you feel as though everything has been lost. There is nothing left but emptiness. To prevent this isolation and to reduce your fear of injury, Dr. Jeffers recommends nurturing your whole life. Giving 100% commitment and acting as if you count in each of your roles is what she refers to as the "Magic Duo."[7]

In an effort to maintain athletic identity, a frequent response to sports injury is substituting activities. You have probably observed the athlete who goes from running to cycling to swimming, always in search of the activity that does not hurt. I did this, though in a different order. When biking hurt my back, I took up running and swimming. When I couldn't do these sports, I went hiking or golfing. I even tried surfing. I was desperate to stay active and to feel like an athlete.

Changing sports will not guard against the devastation of another injury when the list of alternatives has been exhausted. Taking Dr. Jeffers' advice—balancing your life by building on your roles and relationships—reduces your fear and makes you more able to handle whatever life has in store for you. Hopefully, it's not another injury, but if so, you will have the tools to manage it better the next time around.

While I was laid up, I found satisfaction in taking a more active role as a friend, student, hobbyist, sister and teacher. I filled my social calendar with fun events with friends, spent more time in creative pursuits, read about healing and bikes, visited my sister, and began sharing my story with others through blogs. I strove to see my setback as an opportunity for growth in other areas of my life.

The Second Stage of Grief: Anger

This injury isn't going away! You can only deny your injury for so long when you have repeated reminders that something is wrong. Denial is a defense mechanism that shelters us from this truth. There comes a point, however, when you cannot deny the pain any longer, and anger surfaces.

Your rage may appear in small ways that are unrelated to your injury at first. You might have a general sense of being in a bad mood, easily losing your temper and responding more dramatically to everyday stresses with exaggerated actions. These are all signs that you have moved to the next stage of grief. Eventually, your feelings of annoyance and exasperation will be directed at your injury.

As you heard in my story in Chapter 1, I was outraged about my hip injury. I couldn't believe another joint had failed me. I wanted to know why this was happening to me and not other athletes. Why did I continue to suffer recurrent injuries, while my friends and competitors could train on without interruption? I wanted to blame someone or something else for my pain. Were my sports causing my pain? Are sports bad? No. If that were true, nobody would be able to play sports injury-free. Was it my coach's fault? Perhaps. I was self-coaching, and, unlike my dedicated clients who follow my guidance, I didn't always take my own advice. The hard reality, which I didn't want to accept, was that there was something about myself to blame. I couldn't point my finger at an external entity. I had to accept that my physical structure was the culprit of my suffering. This made me furious!

As an athlete, you are very careful about your conditioning. You follow a systematic training plan to optimize fitness and to prevent physical breakdown and injury. As an athlete, you realize the strength of your body is paramount to successful sports performance. With all this focused attention on being in peak shape, I found it to be unbelievable that such a tragic injury could occur in my body. As I introduced in Chapter 1 and will discuss in more detail in coming chapters, my unbalanced body and faulty muscle mechanics were the cause of my pain. Reaching the conclusion that my body was defective, I despised it. I hated my body for being fragile, twisted, and weak, and I hated it for not allowing me to ride my bike.

The Third Stage of Grief: Bargaining

mind

If I'm good, will you make the pain go away? The terminally ill patients of Dr. Kübler-Ross were bargaining for a longer life, usually in secret with God. As Dr. Kübler-Ross explains, "The bargaining is really an attempt to postpone; it has to include a prize offered 'for good behavior,' it also sets a self-imposed 'deadline'."[1] Your bargaining is different from these patients. You are not trying to postpone death, but you are trying to enjoy your life more completely without pain and injury. You may try bargaining with your healthcare providers, universe/religious/spiritual icons, or yourself. I don't know that bargaining works in cases of pain and injury. However, agreements made with yourself to commit to your healing and to take personal responsibility in the process *are* very powerful. Setting goals, which will be discussed shortly, is one way to hold yourself accountable.

The Fourth Stage of Grief: Depression

I can't take it anymore! At this stage, you cannot deny the existence of injury anymore. You have come to terms with your anger and have made your deals with higher powers for healing. Now the sadness sets in. As humans, we are programmed to be more sensitive to negative news. This disposition toward the unfavorable, known as the "Negativity Bias," developed due to the evolutionary necessity of survival. We had to be alert to danger so that we could avoid it and survive.[8] Today, you are not fighting against predators or battling the weather for your life. Much of the stress you experience today is not of a physical nature; rather, it has psychological and social origins.[9] Regardless of the source, your mindset is still programmed to emphasize the adverse aspects of life, predisposing you to anxiety and depression—thanks to your innate "Negativity Bias."

Martin E. P. Seligman, Ph.D., leading authority in positive psychology and director of the Positive Psychology Center at the University of Pennsylvania, has found a link between depression and pessimism.[10] Through using questionnaires, he found the majority of depressed people have a pessimistic explanatory style. Explanatory style is how a person explains the events that happen in his life. It is the tone of one's story. According to Dr. Seligman, pessimists view setbacks as "permanent, pervasive and personal: 'It's going to last forever, it's going to undermine everything, and it's my fault.'"[11]

When injured, a pessimist will blame himself for his injury because he believes it is personal. He thinks he will never recover 100% and will be plagued with the problem forever because he sees the injury as permanent and pervasive. A pessimist views positive events as having the direct opposite causes of negative events. He views positive events as being the result of external forces—not attributable to himself (impersonal); as being unpredictable—never knowing when or why something good happens; and being specific—thinking that good things only happen in limited situations and are not pervasive.[11] Dr. Seligman has found that "pessimists [...] are up to eight times more likely to become depressed when bad events happen."[11]

Regarding healing, pessimists are dependent on a particular person or therapy to make them better. They feel no control over their recovery, presuming the process will be erratic and that there is nothing they can do about it. Consequently, pessimists may be more inclined to abandon their healing process. Dr. Seligman characterizes this reaction to give up and quit as "learned helplessness," which is common in pessimists.[11]

> *I noticed this in myself: I was pessimistic about my pain and hip injury. I thought I had brought it on myself because of negligence, and I reprimanded myself for not taking better care of myself. I put my faith in someone else to heal me and regularly practiced "catastrophic thinking,"[11] assuming that everything I experienced was negative and a sign I wouldn't recover. For example, I once interpreted a canceled appointment by a therapist to mean she had given up on me, when there was actually a much simpler explanation—her child was sick. This tendency to blame myself for a bad event is known as "personalization." It is characteristic of a pessimistic explanatory style.[12]*

In contrast to pessimists are optimists. Optimists, according to Seligman, believe "their setbacks are surmountable, particular to a single problem, and resulting from temporary circumstances or other people."[12] Optimists tend to have better health than pessimists, age well, and may even live longer. Dr. Seligman gives several reasons for this, including a stronger immune system. As I mentioned in the introduction, all of our systems are interconnected. Depression causes changes in the brain and depletes our hormones. These two effects of depression suppress our immune system. Thus, when we are positive—and not depressed—we can better fight off illness. Optimists are also more likely to have better health because they take positive steps to maintain their wellness, and they quickly seek advice when they become ill. They believe their actions matter. Because of that belief, they take responsibility for their health. Because of this take-charge attitude and proactive approach to life, optimists tend to have fewer bad life events. Finally, optimists willingly seek out others in times of need, while pessimists tend to be more passive in gaining help from others. Since social support and nourishing relationships enhance wellness, optimists are healthier.[11] In fact, research has found that optimists also heal faster from athletic injuries than pessimists.

Optimism Aids Healing

A study by Ievleva and Orlick comparing athletes with knee and ankle injuries showed that the optimistic athletes recovered quicker.[13] Along with optimism—positive attitude and outlook—the researchers attributed several factors to enhanced healing, including stress control, social support, goal setting, positive self-talk and mental imagery. Their results found that the fastest healing athletes had higher scores in all of the factors listed above, compared to the slowest healing athletes.[13]

Optimism has also been linked with the personality trait hardiness. Hardiness is attributed to someone who does well in high-stress conditions. For most athletes, having an injury classifies as a high-stress condition. Hardiness is composed of three traits: commitment, control, and challenge. A person exhibiting hardiness is highly committed to her daily activities and always puts forth her best effort. Like optimists, hardy individuals feel that their actions matter and that they have control over their circumstances. When challenges arise, a person gifted in hardiness sees the problem as an opportunity to be overcome, not as a threat.[14]

Researchers Ford, Gordon and Eklund found injured athletes who experienced high stress and were low in optimism and hardiness took longer to heal.[15] They suggested that the athletes who were already tending toward pessimism and who were experiencing high stress lacked the coping skills needed to handle the additional burden of an injury.

Additional research by Grove, Stewart and Gordon (as cited in Pargman, D. [Ed.], 2007), duplicated the finding that pessimists were low in optimism and hardiness. They also discovered that pessimists were low in self-esteem and vigor.[14,16] Their research suggests that the positive qualities—optimism, hardiness, self-esteem and vigor—trend together, similar to the negative personality characteristics—pessimism, depression, anger and tension. Like the other studies mentioned above, these researchers found pessimistic athletes had longer healing times than the optimists following knee surgery.

Based on all of the evidence, it became clear: optimism accelerates recovery. Part of my healing journey, then, included shifting my explanatory style to a more optimistic outlook. *This is possible!* If you consider that optimism is similar to happiness, research has shown that 40% of what determines your happiness level is your intentional activity.[17] These are the choices and behaviors you engage in every day. While 60% of your happiness seems to be determined by two other factors, life circumstances (10%) and genetics (50%), the rest is in your control.[17]

By choosing activities that kept me focused on the positive, I was able to improve my optimism. One of the habits I adopted was writing in a daily gratitude journal. Each evening I would write down what I was thankful for, trying each day to come up with new things to appreciate. I was grateful for my family, a beautiful sunset, my clients, a warm fire, and so on. In addition, I listened to books about optimism and sought out stories of other athletes who had conquered their injuries, like Petria Thomas, an Olympic Australian swimmer who overcame three shoulder and two ankle reconstruction surgeries.[18] I also surrounded myself with optimistic people who provided their support and encouragement. I had to include my husband in the process, so I had him help me recognize and redirect my thinking when I was going into a negative state.

This continual barrage of positive messages helped to nudge my brain over to a more optimistic state. That's not to say I don't still slip into pessimism—I do, but not as often. I am able to view situations without "catastrophizing" and "personalizing" them. I can see other options, not just the worst-case scenario. This has been liberating, not only in my healing but also in many areas of my life.

mind

Setting Recovery Goals

In addition to optimism, research has found that goal setting speeds recovery.[13] As an athlete, you are probably in the habit of setting sports goals—improve your 5K run time, hike a 14-thousand-foot peak, or place in the Top 10 at Nationals. You can apply this same approach to your healing. Obviously, your goals will be very different, but they can be just as challenging and rewarding.

View your recovery as your training. Make a plan. Instead of interval workouts, you will be doing corrective exercises. Rather than meeting for a group workout, you will be scheduling time with therapists and healthcare professionals. Instead of actively practicing your sport, you'll use visualization and other techniques to strengthen your inner game. To improve in your sport, you already practice discipline and dedication with your training. These same strengths can be used to drive your healing.

A word of caution: *Don't overdo it!* I know you really, really want to get better, so you are highly motivated to heal. Recall how I initially experienced greater pain in my healing process. Don't be naive like I was. More is not always better. When your body is vulnerable, this can be destructive. *You can't power through your recovery!* In many cases, the body can't handle it, so it often responds unfavorably. Part of the challenge of the healing process is letting go of this mindset and giving your body what it needs in the form of appropriate treatments with ample rest and recovery. Although it was a difficult lesson for me to learn in my recovery, it was—and still is—extremely important.

When I was hurt, my activities were very limited. Setting goals helped to motivate and focus me. I set the following goals for my physical, mental, emotional and spiritual recovery:

1. Engage my left gluteal muscles
2. Balance my pelvic position
3. Read about and practice exercises to improve my optimism
4. Use my experience to help others through writing
5. Deepen my connections with family and friends

These are general outcome goals, just to get you thinking. Outcome goals are what you want to achieve long-term. To be successful, short-term behavior-focused goals are also necessary. I set weekly behavioral goals to reach my long-term outcome goals. I committed to doing daily corrective exercises for a minimum of 30 minutes, listening to one inspiring book a week to build a positive mental outlook, publishing one blog a month about my healing process, and setting aside time each week to call or get together with friends and family. These goals kept me focused and helped me appreciate the progress I was making toward my long-term outcome goals of ultimately being pain free and returning to sports. Although I couldn't train as I was accustomed to doing, I enjoyed having the familiarity of a structured plan to keep me on track.

When setting your goals, you want to make them "SMART"—Specific, Measurable, Action-based, Realistic and Time-lined.[19] Here's an example of a long-term SMART goal: "Improve my 15-mile run time in the *Jemez Mountain Trail Run* in 2018 by 10 minutes." A short-term goal to support this outcome might be this: "I will run five miles on Tuesday and Saturday this week." Staying focused on even small accomplishments is motivational, but it is easily forgotten if not documented. *Write it down!*

This is also true for physical improvements. Many times I'll ask clients about a prior limitation or discomfort that was previously a huge deal, only to be met with a blank stare. They can't remember the problem at all. Once the issue is resolved or a goal is reached, we tend to forget about it entirely. The human brain has a funny habit of continuously giving attention to what needs to be done and forgetting about what has already been attained. Do you do that? I do. I reach a milestone, and without a pause, I start planning the next steps. This drive to constantly move forward and succeed is why we often fail at recognizing and rewarding ourselves for what we do achieve.

An essential but often overlooked part of the goal-setting process is giving yourself rewards. When you meet a goal, no matter how small, you want to acknowledge your accomplishment. I know, you might feel you should only be rewarded when you reach your long-term outcome goal. But remember, all of the short-term goals add up and will culminate in achieving your desired outcome. I often find that determining the reward is harder than setting the goal. After creating and documenting goals with clients, I often send them home with homework: send me an email that tells me what their rewards will be. Creating rewards can be such a foreign concept for my clients that they cannot come up with anything quickly during our session. This is especially true if the reward is not centered around food. We love to reward ourselves with chocolate! While a food goal is not bad, per se, if it's not in line with a wellness goal—such as giving yourself chocolate for meeting the goal of cutting back on sweets—then obviously it's not much of a reward, as you're actually defeating the goal itself. The reward doesn't have to be big or cost money. I enjoy a long snuggle on the couch with my doggies in front of the fire. You might consider rewarding yourself with spending extra time on a favorite hobby or soaking in a hot bath. Taking time to reward yourself extends the good feelings that accompany success. As you've learned, keeping a positive mental outlook aids recovery, so savor your victories and accelerate your healing.

Creating Your Recovery Vision

Along with setting goals for your recovery, it is important to appreciate the big picture. A recovery vision depicts the end result. It creates a picture of what your ultimate recovery looks and feels like.[20] Your recovery vision goes beyond alleviating the physical pain and incorporates other dimensions of your life. It gives direction for your recovery goals. Creating a recovery vision is an opportunity for you to explore what kind of athlete you want to be once your pain and injury are gone.

A few questions to consider in creating your recovery vision:

What is your mental state upon recovery?
Are you thinking differently—about your body, your sports, your life?
What is your emotional state upon recovery?
Are you feeling differently—about your body, your sports, your life?
What is your physical state upon recovery?
How has your body changed?
How has your perception and attitude toward your body changed?
What is your spiritual state upon recovery?
What is your understanding of the importance of sports in your life?
What is your role as an athlete?
What behaviors are you engaging in regularly—meaning, what tools and skills are you using that you learned during your healing process?
Who are you surrounding yourself with?
What are the characteristics of your physical environment?
How are you expressing yourself to others and being received by them?

You may have more questions to add, but this will get you started. The more details you can provide, the more effective your vision will be. This is your pain-free destination. You want to make it as engaging, vivid, and inviting as you can. The clearer you can see where you are going, the easier it will be to get there.

Although I did not have this exercise to do while injured, I am pleased with where I ended up in my journey. Looking back, my recovery vision would have been something like this: My physical pain is relieved, and my body is strong. My structure is more aligned and functional. I have the tools and confidence to take care of my body. I don't doubt my ability to be active and to stay pain free. I am deeply connected with my body, listening and respecting its needs. My mind is calm, filled with gratitude, and more optimistic. I do not obsess about competition. I enjoy multiple sports, which keeps me balanced. I appreciate my role as an athlete, and I know that my race results do not define my self-worth. I find significance as a person outside of sports. I am surrounded by people who support this balanced approach to athletics and life. I find meaning in my injury by sharing my story and lessons with others.

The Final Stage of Grief: Acceptance

Okay, I can deal with this. Acceptance does not mean you resign yourself to your injury or that you give up hope for pain relief. Rather, acceptance marks a quieting of the internal struggle characteristic of the previous stages of grief—denial, isolation, anger, bargaining, and depression. Your mental and emotional landscape has turned from crashing ocean waves to a calm mountain lake. You may still experience some unrest about your situation, but overall you feel more at peace.

I don't know if we all reach the stage of acceptance with our injury. Just as many people fight death to the end, some of us will fight through our injury, never fully acknowledging it. I understand and empathize with this mentality, as this is how I handled all three of my knee surgeries. I kept pushing through in an attempt to achieve my goal: return to my mountain bike and competition as soon as possible. When my hip failed, I finally accepted and acknowledged my injury. I came to the very difficult realization that if I continued to abuse my body this way, all I could expect in the future was more surgery and pain with less activity and sports. This was an important lesson for me to learn.

When we accept our injury and stop fighting our situation, we start to see more clearly. Strong emotions cloud our vision and lure us into making bad choices. With clarity of mind, you are ready to fully engage in the work required to heal your body. As you start on your journey, I will advise you on strategies that have worked for me and my clients to make your journey easier and more successful. You'll find seven helpful tips in the next chapter.

mind

Summary

The pain of sports injuries goes beyond the physical sensations. It also includes your mental and emotional responses. It is normal to grieve when suffering from a chronic injury that is keeping you from playing. You have experienced a loss. There are five common stages associated with the grief cycle that you may go through: (1) Denial and Isolation, (2) Anger, (3) Bargaining, (4) Depression and (5) Acceptance. However, you may not necessarily experience all stages or neatly go through them in the defined order, and you may visit a stage more than once in the process.

Losing your identity as an athlete due to injury can be extremely difficult on the mind. Sports may be fulfilling some of your emotional needs (such as significance, self-esteem, and belonging). Without athletics you are challenged to find other ways to meet these needs. One approach to solving this is recognizing the other roles you have in life and investing more into these relationships.

Certain life characteristics make dealing with and recovering from a chronic injury easier. Leading a full life with lots of variety and commitment to your different personal roles and having an optimistic and hardy personality have both been found to be beneficial. Setting goals that are based on a vision of the athlete you want to be upon recovery is also a helpful tool shown to aid healing. Allowing yourself to go through and wrestle with the mental and emotional aspects of your recovery, although hard, will build your mental and emotional strength and resilience.

Game Winning Strategies

Additional copies of the fillable charts—life grid, goal and reward tables—are available for download on my website: www.thepfathlete.com/resources.

mind

1. Diversify Your Life

Complete your life grid with all of the roles you assume.

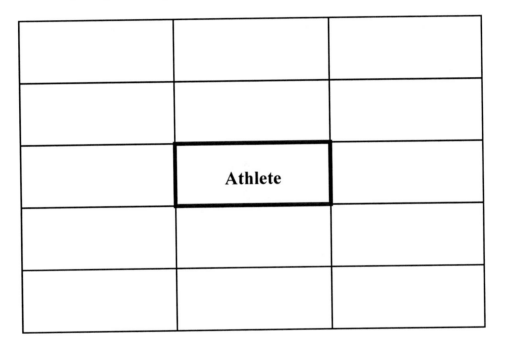

	Athlete	

Circle the role(s) that need more of your energy and attention.

What is one small step you can take in the role(s) you have circled—starting today?

2. Test Your Optimism

Take the Optimism Test on the Authentic Happiness website: www.authentichappiness.sas.upenn.edu/testcenter.

Review the summary report and pick one action item to work on today. Once this has become a habit, maintained for at least three weeks, pick another action item to target.

3. Write Your Recovery Vision

What is your ultimate vision for your recovery?

Use the Recovery Vision questions listed earlier in this chapter as a guide and add any additional ones you have. Then consolidate the information into a few concise sentences.

4. Set Recovery Goals and Rewards

Start with your long-term goals—what you ultimately want.

My Long-Term Goals and Rewards	
Date: _____	
Goal	**Reward**
1.	
2.	
3.	
4.	
5.	

Set short-term (weekly or monthly) goals to support your long-term goals.

My Short-Term Goals and Rewards

Date: _____

Goal	Reward
1.	
2.	
3.	
4.	
5.	

mind

Don't forget to document rewards for each goal, and make sure to give yourself the prize for your accomplishment. *Don't bypass this step, as it's more important than it might seem!*

5. Partner With a Wellness Coach to Speed Your Mental Recovery

As you've read, losing your ability to play sports because of injury or chronic pain can be devastating. You may be experiencing this loss right now. The strong emotions and mental confusion that were discussed in this chapter can be difficult and overwhelming to deal with by yourself. Just talking to someone who "gets you" can bring comfort and the start of healing. *You don't have to do this alone!* Contact The Pain Free Athlete for a free consultation, www.thepfathlete.com/wellness-coaching.

4

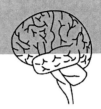

Seven Tips for Your Healing Journey

*H*ealing is an individual journey, unique for each person. I cannot give you a timeline for your recovery, nor can I give you an explicit map directly leading from Point A (injury) to Point B (activity). *I wish I could!* Your injury may be simple to correct or sophisticated in nature, requiring a more advanced therapeutic approach. Along your path from pain to wellness, there may be some trial and error, setbacks and frustration. You may want to give up, or you might lose faith in yourself and your body. Be assured, you will reach your pain-free destination. It may take longer than you think, and it might be harder than you want, but you will get there.

As I went through my holistic healing journey and watched my clients go through theirs, I have observed common mistakes and have learned what aids recovery. In this chapter, I will share these lessons I've learned. Here are seven helpful and interrelated tips for your recovery.

Tip 1: Avoid Mind and Body Overload

When I was hurting, I sought out opinions and treatments from many professionals—too many, in fact. I was in pain, desperate for relief, and wanted the quickest path back to my sports. It didn't work. I was overwhelmed and lacked commitment to anything, so I didn't get better. Today, I see my clients repeating my frantic, unproductive search. They'll spend hours looking up their condition on the internet, sometimes gleaning information from unreliable sources, which only adds to their panic. Yes, you want to be informed and take an active role in your health care, but there is a point where you can go too far and become overloaded. Obsessively chasing "a cure" that probably doesn't exist is not healthy and only keeps you focused on your ailments. The more we give our time, attention and energy to what is wrong with us, the more our health problems grow. This is how the law of attraction works: "Like attracts like. What that means in simple terms for your life is: what you give out, you receive back."[1] Focus on the difficulties of your situation, and expect more difficulties to arise.

Upon seeking abundant sources of information for guidance, there are bound to be contradictions. One therapist tells you to do this, while the chiropractor tells you not to do this, but to do that. Then, the acupuncturist has another idea, the doctor offers a different opinion, and the articles online don't agree. So, what do you do? Some clients become paralyzed and don't do anything, while others try to do it all, not knowing if anything is worth their time and money, and not knowing if anything is even helping.

Your mind gets overloaded—mentally and emotionally—when you acquire too much intellectual information. Also, your body gets over-loaded—physically—when you try too many healing treatments. Your brain and body can only absorb so much information and stimuli. When you're training for cardiovascular sports, you can only do so many high-intensity intervals in a week, month and season; similarly, your body can only do so many rehabilitative exercises or endure so much bodywork when trying to recover. With training and rehabilitation, there comes a point of diminishing returns, where doing more leads to a reduction in gains as well as possible setbacks and injury. My client, Jaqueline, experienced a major backslide in her recovery by doing too much.

Desperate to heal, Jaqueline thought that addressing her recovery with a multifaceted approach of bodywork and therapy activities was going to do better than just one at a time. For example, she was having weekly deep-tissue bioelectric massages, bi-weekly myofascial release treatments, weekly acupuncture sessions, and weekly physical therapy appointments. She was also performing self-myofascial release with a foam roller or therapy balls, conducting posture and physical therapy exercises, and walking on the treadmill daily. The combination of all her well-intentioned, multiple treatments resulted in her body responding with a dramatic increase—not a decrease—in her pain. Basically, her body was telling her to back off. Her over-zealous approach ultimately delayed her healing, as she had to stop and go back to a no-activity regimen. She had to start from ground zero.

More is not always better! You'll need to pace yourself through your healing. The process cannot be rushed or forced, as Jaqueline found out when her efforts backfired. My advice is to identify a few credible sources for information and to stick with those. You'll also want to limit the number of healthcare professionals you have assisting in your recovery at any one time. Eliminating chronic pain can require integrating various healing approaches, and you will want a team of people whom you know, like, and trust by your side throughout your journey.

mind

Tip 2: Establish Your Healing Team

As an injured athlete, you can pick anyone to be on your healing team, so only choose the best. You want to select people you respect and feel a close connection with. You want to know that your best interests and recovery are as high a priority for your healthcare provider as they are for you. Avoid making the mistake of using a particular doctor or therapist just because your friend did or because the person has come highly recommended. It is essential that you feel comfortable and relaxed with your provider. You are entering into a patient/client-provider relationship where personal information will be shared, and you must feel you can be open and honest. If not, your healing will be compromised and possibly delayed—or not attained at all. The patient/client-healthcare provider relationship has a strong influence on your recovery outcome. In her book, *Mind Over Medicine,* Dr. Lissa Rankin discusses the power of nurturing care. She explains that having a healthcare professional who is nurturing, trusting and reassuring makes you feel better immediately because your stress declines and your relaxation response is induced, which increases your body's ability to heal itself.[2]

It is okay to remove a healthcare professional from your team. Sometimes things just don't work out. You may find there is a personality conflict or a problem with the healing approach. In the end, *you* are responsible for *your* recovery. Your team is there to provide support and to give guidance, but *you* have the final say in the healing path followed. If a procedure or therapy is being recommended that doesn't seem right to you, respect your inner wisdom and go elsewhere. The goal of any good and ethical healthcare provider is your recovery. As a coach myself, I only work with clients I believe will benefit from my interventions. If it's not a good client-coach match, I will offer referrals to other providers. A healthcare provider with this mentality will not be upset or offended when taken off the team roster. Rather, it is a learning opportunity for her to understand why you didn't improve. It helps her to refine her techniques and do better with the next person. These professionals also realize that their tools are not going to work for everyone; another therapeutic approach might be more appropriate for you than what they can offer.

Your team can be made up of a wide variety of practitioners. The key is that the people you select fit your requirements—people that you respect, know, like, have a connection with, and trust. As you progress along your holistic healing journey, your team may change. At the time of my hip surgery, my team members included an orthopedic surgeon, a physical therapist, a chiropractor and a massage therapist. Following surgery, I delved into more complementary medicine treatments and made substitutions and additions to my team, including an Egoscue Method® therapist, an acupuncturist/herbalist, an Alexander Technique® instructor, a structural integration and visceral manipulation bodyworker, an optometrist, an orthodontist, and various physical therapists. Although not directly on my team, I also worked with a Chi Running® instructor, an Active Isolated Stretching® practitioner, a yoga instructor, a Reiki therapist, a MELT Method® instructor, and a Pilates instructor during my healing. No, I didn't work with all of these people and methods at the same time; in fact, I tried them all but kept only those that benefitted me the most. If you are drawn to try something and feel it may help, go for it—but beware of overwhelming your systems. When expanding your treatment options this way, you are in control and are not obligated to continue any approach or to remain in contact with any particular healthcare professional if it is not a fit for you. And, you may find that an additional or different technique provides the relief you seek.

Experimenting with different therapeutic modalities is part of the healing journey. After you try something a time or two, you'll know if it resonates with you. I only did several of the techniques listed above less than a handful of times. You'll need to be selective about what you choose to do in order to avoid overload by keeping your team roster short. The important thing is that you surround yourself with the best healthcare professionals for you, believe in your treatment, and fully commit to the process.

Tip 3: Believe and Commit to Your Healing Approach

Your healing is ultimately up to you. Along your journey you will seek out professionals to assist you, and you will gain valuable knowledge. However, in the end, you have control and will make the decisions about which treatments to pursue. When making those hard choices, it is important that you have confidence and trust in the process and the people supporting you. The treatment plan you follow should make intellectual sense, as your mind has to buy into what you are doing with your body. If you doubt what you are doing, you will likely fail. Therefore, you must have an emotional connection to your healing approach. It needs to feel "right." That's how it was for me with Egoscue® posture alignment therapy.

In the beginning, I was skeptical about the Egoscue Method®.[3] My first introduction to the method was from a personal training client who loaned me Pete Egoscue's Pain Free book.[4] I flipped through the book and skipped right to the hip exercises section without reading a word of the chapter itself. As I did the program, I highly doubted something so simple could be effective and help me. Not surprisingly, I didn't notice an instant change in my pain from the exercises, and I promptly dropped the approach.

When my massage therapist Susan urged me to give the Egoscue Method® a try the following year, I smiled and graciously accepted her gift: my own copy of Pain Free.[4] Despite her budding enthusiasm about the approach and her faith that it would help me, I quickly deposited the book on my shelf without a glance when I returned home. Been there, done that. Several months later, when I was feeling desperate, still in pain, and running out of treatment options, I reached for the book. Of course, I didn't use the book as suggested—which was to read the first three chapters, and then go to your pain area—but, rather, I jumped right into completely reading the chapter on hips (not just the section on hip exercises as I had previously done). Yikes! The book explained how some hip replacements are unnecessary; it stated that many people still have pain after the invasive procedure due to musculoskeletal dysfunctions. And, if these imbalances aren't corrected, the other hip or the knees can also be affected.[4]

mind

The knees! My left one was already seriously impaired and on its way to needing replacement. Also shocking was the statement, "cartilage will regenerate—but only if it is allowed to."[4] What? I had been told the opposite and to curtail rigorous, pounding activities, like running, that would further the breakdown of these delicate tissues. The final blow was the description of Osteoarthritis as "a symptom of joint misalignment."[4]

I was taken aback and uncertain about these outrageous claims that defied all the guidance and information I had read, heard, or received first-hand from medical professionals until this point. However, I wanted to believe that the Egoscue Method® would work for me. And with an open and hopeful attitude, I started the hip program exercises again. My mindset had been changed, and I was fully committed to the process. I sought out a therapist in Albuquerque (two hours from my home) to work with me individually and enrolled in the training program to become certified in the Egoscue Method®. I went all in, and guess what? This time it worked! More details to come in Chapters 6 and 8.

Tip 4: Don't Become Your Diagnosis

Osteoarthritis, stenosis, tendonitis, sciatica, bursitis—these are all just fancy words used to label and categorize your pain. A diagnosis is merely a word used by medical professionals and logged on insurance forms for reimbursement. The pain was the same before, and it is the same after attaching this noun to it. The way you respond to this label in body, mind and spirit, however, is critical and will dictate your recovery.

After my left hip arthroscopic surgery in 2007, I was diagnosed with severe (grade 4) bone-on-bone osteoarthritis (OA). I was 38. When my doctor and I parted, his last words were, "I'll see you in 15 years for your hip replacement." Too young for a joint replacement, I was advised to reduce my activity level and avoid any movements that hurt. When the pain was excruciating enough, and my activity limited enough, I would be considered for a new artificial hip.

Receiving a formal diagnosis of any kind makes your heart sink. Now you have a big, ugly word to attach to your pain and by which to label yourself. I have arthritis. I am an arthritis sufferer! I can now commiserate with others who share my same condition. I belong to a group! Some people (yes, like me) proudly stand behind their diagnosis, finally having something definitive to point to as the cause of the pain. Soon after my diagnosis, I picked up a copy of the magazine Arthritis Today, bought a book on alternative therapies for arthritis, looked into support groups and talked to others who shared my plight. I was resigned and preparing to surrender to my disease.

Until . . . I met with an Egoscue Method® therapist, whose reaction to my arthritis story was, "So you have a little inflammation in your hip?" Whoa! A little inflammation? No, I have this serious life-changing condition that is never going away. I had attached myself to this diagnosis and had made a big deal of it. I was offended! I thought my OA was something severe. I was disconcerted by his dismissive and belittling comment and didn't know how to respond. Some time later, another Egoscue Method® therapist, Mark, told me that I wore my OA diagnosis on my sleeve for everyone to see and admire. I didn't know I was portraying myself that way, nor did I want to.

These Egoscue Method® therapists didn't mess around. They called me out on my self-pity party. I was stuck in the depression stage of the grief cycle, and they were challenging me to move on. It was a turning point for me. As Mark and I continued our conversation, he asked me why I didn't run. I replied, "I was told not to run by my doctor; running is bad and will wear out my hip faster." Mark smiled, as I'm sure he had heard this excuse many times before. After watching me do my Egoscue® posture exercises, and after performing a few hip mobility and strength tests, he stated that I had better hip function than nearly all of the hip patients he had treated. He thought my hip was sound, and if I continued with my therapy, I shouldn't need a replacement. He also said that I should be fine to run. So, I did.

Mark's message was clear: You can do more than you think. You are holding yourself back from reaching your potential by believing otherwise. How many of us limit ourselves in our minds? We buy into the accepted beliefs about what someone with arthritis, or any other medical diagnosis, can or cannot do.

This experience illustrates how our mental and emotional attitudes towards our diagnosis can influence the direction of our healing. It also shows how we can limit ourselves and our healing potential with faulty beliefs. If I hadn't had these tough encounters where my thinking was challenged, I may have never run again. I probably would have acquiesced to the doctor's prediction of gradually increasing pain and a steady decline in my athletic ability. I am ever thankful for being pushed outside my comfort zone to consider another possibility for my life.

I was lucky. Many people are not as fortunate. When told by their medical provider to avoid activities or to have risky surgeries, they quietly comply, often giving up years of quality life. As a coach, I strive to challenge and empower my clients, just as I was challenged and empowered during my therapy. I encourage my clients not to settle for the dire future predictions they have been given. I emphasize my belief in the power of the body to heal and rejuvenate, regardless of age.

Close relationships and deep connections with others are vital during your healing journey. Not only can these people push you to improve, but they can also provide the support and encouragement you need during the hard times.

Tip 5: Find Support Wherever You Can

I was fortunate to have a wonderful team in my corner when I was injured and at my worst: a loving husband, an understanding family, and caring friends. My best source of support and motivation, though, was Coral, my beloved yellow Labrador Retriever. She and her older sister Sandy, also a yellow Lab, brought great joy to my life. Shortly after Coral turned one, she had knee surgery. It wasn't clear if she had a birth defect or had suffered an accident, but somehow she chipped her left kneecap. Only a week after Coral had her knee repair procedure, I had the first arthroscopic surgery on my left knee. Over 15 years of gymnastics and hundreds of miles on the bike seemed to have taken its toll on my cartilage and joint tissues.

As recovery companions, Coral and I would rest on the bed in a daze from our pain medications while we healed. Not wanting to be left out, Sandy joined us, too, though she seemed bored by the whole thing. Sandy tried to motivate us to move and play but got nowhere for her efforts. She would rush the door when my husband, Ken, arrived home, overjoyed to have someone with energy around to take her out for a game of fetch.

Within a few days, Coral and I were up and about, again much to Sandy's relief. I took to slow, stationary bike rides for my recovery. Coral, on the other hand, tried to walk, run and jump on her rebuilt knee without delay. Holding her back and limiting her movement to allow full recovery was impossible for Ken and me. She was a dog. She didn't know any better, and she was ready to go.

Oh, how I envied Coral's quick return and free will toward her activities. My recovery was not as complete. Instead of enjoying a new lease on life, I was told to be careful with my body and activities to avoid further damage to my cartilage. I was advised that it would only be a matter of time before my knee was full of arthritis, and I shouldn't do anything to accelerate the process. For someone who bounced out of her crib as an infant, took up tumbling at five years old, played all the sports made available to her, had been a competitive gymnast, loved cross-country skiing, and was on her way to becoming an elite mountain biker, this was devastating news. Fortunately, I could still bike, so I pedaled on, but with increased caution. The voice in the back of my mind continuously warning me of danger and impending doom if I did too much.

Alternatively, Coral lacked any fear of re-injury. One day, as we were pulling up to a reservoir to take the dogs for a swim, Coral leaped from the back of the truck and through the camper shell's window screen before we had even parked. This was a drop to the ground of over four feet. She darted straight for the water to retrieve a fisherman's bobber, which must have looked like an irresistible red ball to her eyes.

How do you tell a dog not to run and jump? You don't! The ironic thing is, Coral's cavalier attitude and refusal to give in to her injury worked for her, and she had no more knee incidents. For me, however, I would have two more surgeries on my left knee.

mind

73

Over Memorial Day weekend in 2007, Coral's life changed, as did mine. At seven and a half, Coral became paralyzed in her hind end from pouncing too aggressively on a tennis ball during a game of fetch. Our bounding, zestful dog had become a special needs dog with a neurological disorder after a single dive on a tennis ball. With my recurrent knee surgeries, I began to wonder if I would have the same fate. Play hard, give it everything you have, 125%, and you'll end up with a serious, permanent injury. Was that going to be my future, too?

You may call this a self-fulfilling prophecy because, as it would happen, at about the same time Coral became paralyzed, I had a sudden change in my ability to move. Debilitating back pain made it impossible for me to sit on my bike and reach forward to the handlebars. Also, I had this ache in my hip that wouldn't abate. One day I was a professional mountain bike racer, and the next, I was unable to bend over and pick up a pen off the floor or walk without a limp. Toward the end of that summer, I had my hip surgery. Coral and I, once again, were recovery partners.

Our healing required many specialists, alternative approaches, patience, dedication, and daily exercise. Coral showed me how to manage my injury with grace and dignity. Lacking higher cognitive function, Coral was not plagued with a mind that could regret, worry about others' opinions, lose confidence, or doubt her abilities. Though she might have been able to experience emotions such as distress, she didn't show any signs.[5] She maintained her incredible drive and will to live. Her staggering gait and occasional falls didn't slow her down. Through all her days, she continued to run after tennis balls and barked at dogs twice her size, chasing them until she collapsed.

Coral touched the lives of many, being referred to as a wonder dog, amazing, super dog and "the little dog that could." Coral's strength of character kept me going and smiling when I hurt, felt sorry for myself, and wanted to quit. She was an inspirational and motivating role model. I was lucky to have her at my side during my recovery.

Coral was a great canine therapist who taught me many things about healing and recovery. Here are five lessons that I learned from her.

CORAL'S LESSON #1

Daily therapy keeps you moving—move it or lose it

Immediately after Coral's accident, and for several years following, she went to physical therapy, exercising on the underwater treadmill. She also did an obstacle course and daily leash walks to maintain her strength and improve her coordination. She was one of my first clients. When she missed her therapy, there was a noticeable decline in her function.

Similarly, when I skip my morning posture routine, I can feel the difference. It is essential that I keep my body aligned and muscles limber and strong, as it enables me to continue participating in the sports I most enjoy. It's just another way that I take care of my health, like brushing my teeth. Performing daily posture exercises is how I keep my body systems in good alignment and functioning optimally.

CORAL'S LESSON #2

It's okay to accept help from others—swallow your ego and be vulnerable

When fatigued, Coral could only take a few steps without collapsing. To aid her and to relieve the work in her rear, I'd place a support strap under her belly. With this assistance, her pace quickened, and she'd be fired up to keep going. She really seemed to appreciate the help.

In many areas of my life, I wanted to do everything myself without asking for help. I felt that if I did reach out to others, I would be seen as weak. This limiting belief has been hard to break. My hip injury changed this; I couldn't do it alone like I had with my past knee surgeries. Although initially hesitant, I quickly found many supportive resources. People want to help you. It is their calling, just as it is now mine. Building a trusted team around me has been essential in my healing.

mind

CORAL'S LESSON #3

> Stay focused on what you want—not on what you've lost
>
> Dogs narrow in on what they want—ball, ball, ball! When Coral had a tennis ball, she could be hard to distract, even with food. She knew what she wanted and could not be deterred.
>
> When injured, I found it hard to imagine another reality and obsessed about not being able to ride my bike. I became absorbed in my pain and limitations, endlessly fearing I would never get better. With time, I realized that directing my energy into what I couldn't do while injured was greatly slowing my healing. Shifting my thoughts and actions to what was within my abilities, focusing on what I could do, was empowering and rewarding.

CORAL'S LESSON #4

> Believe in yourself, and be hopeful about the future
>
> Regardless of how many times Coral fell down, she demonstrated the same determination and enthusiasm to get back up on her feet, again and again. Every time she tried to stand, she'd tirelessly reach and jump her front paws forward so she could maneuver her back side up and get a good grip with her doggie booties. *Triumph!*
>
> Being human, it is easy to feel defeated with repeated failures. We begin to second guess, lose momentum, and even give up. To Coral, a slip was merely a temporary setback to be overcome. She didn't doubt. She may have struggled; she may have had to try a few times; but she persisted in reaching her goal.

CORAL'S LESSON #5

> Never give up the things you love—*Chase the ball!*

Coral never stopped playing fetch. It was a part of her; it was what she did that brought her extreme pleasure. After her accident, the only thing that changed was the intensity with which she played. No longer did I whack the tennis ball with a racket to gain maximum distance for her to retrieve. Now we played a more gentle game of catch, throwing short lobs in the front yard. She still had a great time!

It was hard for me to get back on the mountain bike after my hip surgery. After all, when a person has been good at something, she wants and expects to reach that level again—quickly. It was difficult for me to let go of that image of myself and not feel inadequate on the bike. Post injury, I did not ride as much as before—I could no longer do 24-hour solo races—but when I got back on my bike, I remembered how fun it was and truly enjoyed the experience.

mind

Tip 6: Find Healthy, Non-Movement Techniques to Manage Stress

Injuries raise your stress level. Looking back at the previous tips, each of these could be a source of stress. Your stress may escalate because you have overloaded your mind or body with stimuli; you feel you have to heal all alone; you cannot find a treatment approach you believe in; you have strongly attached to your diagnosis; and you lack positive social support. When I initially meet with a new client, I ask about stress levels and coping mechanisms. If the client's only form of stress management is exercise, it raises a red flag for me. These clients, lacking other coping resources, tend to have a harder time during recovery than clients with a broader approach to reducing stress. Helping them find other forms of stress management is a priority for me to aid their healing process.

Managing stress without moving can be a challenge. It was for me. I have never been one to sit still. I have been on the move since I was young. With this early introduction to movement, it became my automatic, unconscious stress reliever. I hadn't learned any other way to manage stress. When my wellness coaching mentor asked me to stop and be with my breath for five minutes, I loudly protested, telling her I didn't have time for that. What I was really saying was that I didn't value being still. *I had a lot to learn!*

How can you best manage your escalating stress in a positive, non-destructive way? For some, it is easy to fall into the routine of emotional eating to soothe yourself or drinking alcohol for escape. Neither of these is a positive, long-term strategy. Both will undermine your performance once your pain is gone. You may have to stretch yourself to try some new things to calm your mind. I went back to my mentor's advice about slowing down and breathing, and I even joined a meditation group. Every week we would gather to learn new techniques and take advantage of the group energy to deepen our individual, daily practice. I also tried self-hypnosis audio recordings, which I found uplifting and relaxing.

Biofeedback was another tool I used to lower my stress. While hooked up to a machine, I received instant feedback about my level of anxiety through a change in sound. I controlled the volume and frequency of the sound through my physiology. A softer and slower sound indicated a state of relaxation. I actually became pretty good at it, being able to drop into a peaceful state quicker each time. When I would feel myself become stressed about my injury, I could use this skill to help me relax and maintain control, not allowing myself to get stuck in earlier stages of the grief cycle—isolation, anger, or depression.

You'll need to find your own way to manage stress. You might explore music, reading, writing, socializing, journaling, cooking, baths, crafts—all the things you enjoy but do not have time to do when you are training. These are now great activities to help with stress management. View this as a temporary shift of your energy focus, but consider keeping these new stress management techniques alive even after you resume sports.

After I started playing again, I continued to write, read, take relaxing baths, spend more time with friends and family, sit quietly while focusing on my breathing, and cook more often with my husband. These practices have helped me to maintain balance in my life; they have allowed for the recovery time that I had previously denied myself. Since implementing these practices, I have not had another serious injury or surgery. If this were to happen, though, I now have a better toolkit to handle the stressors that come with these situations.

Through these regular nurturing practices, I have increased my experience of positive emotions and have built greater resilience to any future negative life events, such as another injury or a recurrence of chronic pain. This is in accordance with the "broaden-and-build theory" of positive emotions, introduced by Barbara Fredrickson, Ph.D., Kenan Distinguished Psychology Professor and lead investigator in "Positive Emotions" at the University of North Carolina at Chapel Hill.[6] She states that positive emotions expand our outlook, letting us see more possibilities and the big picture. Additionally, her studies have shown that positive emotions build our emotional reserves and increase our ability to come back from adversity,[6] such as an athletic injury.

mind

Tip 7: Acknowledge and Embrace What You Can Do

One strategy that helped me to develop a more cheerful outlook was to focus on what I *could* do. When injured, I tended to notice only what had been taken from me: riding my bike. I was blind to all of the activities that I could do that were still available to me. I couldn't appreciate other pain-free movements that I could perform, nor could I be grateful for what was possible. All I wanted to do, all I cared about, was riding my bike. I couldn't let go of this deprivation.

During my recovery, I learned there were *many* things I could do. Physically, I could hike, rock climb, swim, golf, stretch, and take my beloved dogs for walks. I even learned to surf, with my sister's guidance, while off the bike. I had been so obsessed about cycling and racing that I believed nothing else could exist outside of this self-defined world. *I was wrong!* I just didn't value the other sports and activities that I *could* do as much as I valued cycling, and therefore, I discounted their importance. I needed to learn to be thankful for what was possible and what I was capable of doing. Note the following story about how I overcame my negative association (discussed in Chapter 2) with the pool and swimming.

Whenever I'm injured, I always take to the pool—swimming, aqua jogging, aqua walking, and exercises with the noodle. Over the course of my many injuries, I had developed a strong aversion to the aquatic center. "The Blue Whale," as our Los Alamos community pool is called, became associated with pain and injury. It was the place I had to go to when I couldn't do what I really wanted to do. My perception was that water exercise was boring, repetitive, inside, cold, smelly, crowded, and just no fun at all. But it was all I could do, so I went—when I tore my quad, after my knee surgeries, and to recover from my hip arthroscopic surgery. As soon as I felt well enough to be outside doing anything else, I quickly fled from the pool and stayed far away.

To make swimming more bearable, I used the ever-popular technique of distraction. There is a reason health clubs are lined with TVs and blare loud music. One of my clients loaned me an aqua mp3 player. Cool! Now I could listen to tunes while I turned my strokes. I swam longer than ever as I hummed to the Reggae beat. Unfortunately, the loan ended, and I had to give the nifty set-up back. I missed the music, something I commonly used while exercising, so I decided to buy my own equipment. I didn't want to spend much since I wouldn't be swimming for long, so I bought a "water proof" holder for my mp3 player. It was more involved than the cool goggle mounts I had borrowed. My set-up had long cords and a bulky container I had to clip to my suit. All the preparations were worth the hassle, though, and I was soon swishing through the water to my favorite 80's tunes. This only lasted for about a week—at which time my mp3 player flooded, due to operator error in the sealing process. Now what?

I was back to swimming in silence. Since it looked like swimming was going to be part of my life for a while, as my hip injury was slow to recover, I thought maybe it was time for a truce between me and swimming. It was time to stop fighting it. I needed to change my attitude and to appreciate swimming for the activity that it is; I needed to be thankful I could do it. I have always enjoyed sports that are dependent on technique for success—Nordic skiing, gymnastics, running, golf, mountain biking—and swimming has a complex technique. I read Total Immersion, a guide for making swimming a "mindful fluid movement."[7] This book offered swimming technique pointers and drills, which I practiced in the pool. I began focusing on what my position was in the water, how to move my hands to gain momentum, and where the kick originated. I began to feel the water going over my body and to feel connected with my sensations. With my new appreciation for the swimming stroke, I didn't loathe going to the pool anymore. I found that paying attention to technique was challenging, and I was motivated to improve. I had discovered a way to enjoy and gain satisfaction while swimming, and I was happier for it. Finally, I had learned gratitude for one of the activities that I could do.

This chapter was intended to give you some tips for your holistic healing journey. It provided ideas on what to do and what to avoid as you go through your process. Next, you'll start to define your course for recovery, considering the options for your treatment.

mind

Summary

This chapter provided seven tips for your recovery.

Tip 1: Avoid Mind and Body Overload
Limit the amount of information you read on your condition and number of treatments you try simultaneously.

Tip 2: Establish Your Healing Team
Surround yourself with a small group of professionals that you know, like and trust, and that care as much as you do about your recovery.

Tip 3: Believe and Commit to Your Healing Approach
To be successful, you cannot doubt and must apply yourself fully to the path you choose for your treatment.

Tip 4: Don't Become Your Diagnosis
A word does not change what you feel, nor does it reduce your possibility for healing and regaining your athletic lifestyle.

Tip 5: Find Support Wherever You Can
People (and animals) want to take care of and comfort you during your recovery, so seek them out and let them help you.

Tip 6: Find Healthy, Non-Movement Techniques to Manage Stress
Calming the nervous system is essential to healing. Find and stick with a relaxing practice that brings you peace.

Tip 7: Acknowledge and Embrace What You Can Do
Although it might be hard to recognize, there are activities you can do while injured. Give your attention and appreciation to these pursuits.

Your road to recovery may not always be smooth, but if you keep your eye on the pain-free destination ahead, you will get there. These tips will make your journey easier.

Game Winning Strategies

1. Prepare for Your Healing Journey

Listed below are journal questions for each tip. You may find you are doing great in some areas but have room for improvement in others. Feel free to skip questions that don't apply to you. For the questions where you find work is needed, also write the first simple step you can take toward success.

mind

Tip 1: Avoid Mind and Body Overload
How are you gathering information about your condition?
How many sources are you consulting?
Do you trust them all?
Do you need to limit your sources to avoid overload?
What would you cut out?
How many body therapies are you doing simultaneously?
Is the amount appropriate, or do you need to make additions, reductions or changes?

Tip 2: Establish Your Healing Team
Who is on your healing team?
Do you know, like and trust everyone on your roster?
Do you need to make cuts to your team?
Do you feel there are gaps in your care?
If so, who should be added?

Tip 3: Believe and Commit to Your Healing Approach
Are you confident in your healing approach?
Are you consistently doing the actions you believe will aid your recovery?
If not, what needs to change?

Tip 4: Don't Become Your Diagnosis
Are you attached to your diagnosis, defining yourself by it?
If so, how can you distance yourself from this label?

Tip 5: Find Support Wherever You Can
Where are you finding support during your healing?
Do you have adequate assistance and encouragement for your healing journey?
Where might you gain more allies?
What can you learn from your role models and those around you?

Tip 6: Find Healthy, Non-Movement Techniques to Manage Stress
What techniques are you using to manage the stress that comes with being injured?
Are your approaches positive and supportive of your return to sports?
Are you doing enough?
Is what you are doing effective for you?
Do you need to find more or other tools?

Tip 7: Acknowledge and Embrace What You Can Do
What can you physically do?
Are you doing those things or lamenting your losses?
What is it going to take to turn your attention away from your limitations and onto your abilities?
Do you appreciate the sports and activities you can do?
How can you develop more gratitude for these activities?

2. <u>Define Your Own Tips</u>

In this chapter I shared with you what I have learned about the healing journey, but there is always room for more and different options.

Reflecting on what you have read, combined with your previous experiences and understanding, what additional tips would you add to what I have provided?

I encourage you to revisit this question as you progress along your journey and when you reach your pain-free destination. Your answers will provide valuable insight in the future if you or anyone near you needs healing.

mind

5

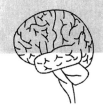

Treating Your Injury

*W*hen injured, many of us follow the same medical path to find relief. We start by scheduling an appointment with our doctor. Or, if the injury is more severe, we don't wait for office hours: we go directly to the urgent care clinic or the emergency room. The healthcare provider assesses the damage, often taking an X-ray or performing other medical tests, and determines the next course of action. Hopefully, this begins with a conservative protocol. If this does not soothe the pain, you may be referred to an orthopedic surgeon. Within the standard orthopedic's tool box are pills, needles for injections, scalpels for surgery, and a referral pad for physical therapy. At the end of this medical cycle, the result should be that you, the athlete, are healed and ready to get back into the game. You may have taken this route. I did. Unfortunately, for me, it didn't provide the healing I wanted. I was still in pain after all the procedures and physical therapy was done. *Now what?*

This chapter will help you to answer that question. The first thing to appreciate about how you approach your healing is that your decisions are dependent on your mindset, which is shaped by three factors: (1) your previous experiences: you may consider what has previously worked for you or for others you know with your current or similar condition, (2) your beliefs: you may select a healing strategy based on what you believe your body needs to heal, and (3) your environment: you may seek advice from the people closest to you, in your immediate environment—family, doctors, friends, therapists, etc. In most cases you will be highly influenced by all of these factors and will make a decision in line with your mindset.

Since the treatment path you choose is the result of many cognitive variables, some of which you may not be aware of, this chapter brings these to the surface for you to examine. Specifically, I will target the second factor in your treatment decision: your beliefs about healing. This chapter gives you an alternative direction to consider for your recovery. Let's start sorting out how you should treat your injury and pain by looking at my client Helen's story.

Choosing a Treatment Path

Helen, whom you first met in Chapter 2 when discussing the wide-reaching effects of pain, explains the process she went through in choosing her treatment path.

I'm 36. I shouldn't be having back pain. Yet I did, and it was truly debilitating. My co-workers would walk by my cubicle, see me lying on the floor, and have a moment of panic that I had collapsed and was unconscious. When it was really bad, I went out to my car and laid down so I wouldn't be bothered. I sent a chat to a friend: "You will never guess where I am!" She replied, "Santa Fe? Alaska? Hawaii?" "No, lying in the backseat of my car at the grocery store, waiting for the ibuprofen to kick in."

My pain started in January, after an overzealous basement clean-out project with too much lifting and bending over. A hike up the ski hill with skins on my skis really set the downward trend in motion. Pretty soon my ski outings were limited to cross country, with multiple stops to lie down and "ice" my back.

I went to the doctor, had massages, went to a physical therapist (PT), and reconnected with Jessica for posture therapy. I tried an SI [sacroiliac] belt, exercises, stretches, ice, heat, and rest. It got to the point where I couldn't sit, and the heavy-duty painkiller Tramadol was really the only thing that was touching the pain.

In mid-April, I woke up with the back of my right calf numb. The next day I was limping, and the numbness and pain extended all the way down the back of my leg and into my foot. This scared me. An MRI [Magnetic Resonance Imaging] revealed that I had a herniated disk at L5/S1. Off I went to a neurosurgeon, who recommended a microdiscectomy to remove the portion of the disk that was pushing on the nerve. I cried. I had never had any kind of surgery before, let alone back surgery! I did not choose surgery easily. I got a second opinion with another doctor (who did not recommend surgery as strongly). I went back to my primary care doctor. I made pros and cons lists. I talked with friends and acquaintances. In the end, I put my trust in my primary care doctor who said, "I'm so sure this will make you better." I needed to hear that. Only because I had an established relationship with her and trusted her was I able to take such a leap.

Other factors that contributed to my decision were the statistics for the success rate for this kind of surgery (well over 90%). Yes, it was back surgery, but a relatively minor one. The risks of not doing surgery were also scary… it could start to affect my bladder control. My husband and I were starting to realize that we did want to have children, and a pregnancy in that condition would make the back pain worse, and surgery would not be an option.

It is now a year to the day that I received my herniated disk diagnosis, and my back is doing great! I even just returned from a mountain bike ride. The recovery that I had dreaded so much was not as bad as I feared. I got a lot of reading done, and I learned that I can handle some down time. I did my PT exercises, I kept working with Jessica on posture alignment, and I walked a lot. It seemed like an eternity until I could get on my bike again in August. When August came, I realized I was content being able to walk and swim pain free. The numbness took longer to go away. I was told it may never go away, but gradually it did.

My co-workers now ask me, "How's your back doing?" and I find myself forgetting that I had back surgery! Just as my aunt encouraged me in the lowest moments, a year from now you will look back on this as just a blip.

Surgery was the right choice for Helen. She believed it would work; she had experiences from others and evidence that it would work; and many people in her environment—friends, family, healthcare providers—also believed it would work. Consequently, it did, and she is doing great, getting stronger every time I see her.

I am not opposed to surgery. While some argue that complementary approaches can fix all, I do not subscribe to this thinking. I would be a hypocrite if I did, considering my long list of operations. Surgery has its place; we are fortunate to have access to these inventive procedures for healing. Drastic measures like surgery, though, shouldn't be the first choice, nor should they be taken lightly or rushed.

The benefits of surgery span the physical, mental, emotional, and spiritual. When Helen was diagnosed with a herniated disc, I asked her if she would ever have confidence in her back if she didn't have the surgery. She quickly said, *"No."* She had seen the MRI of her extruded disc material pushing on her nerve and had felt the consequent numbness, tingling, and pain. Without removing the offending material, she didn't think complete recovery would be possible. She believed her back would always be vulnerable to re-injury. In addition to this mental stress, Helen was also feeling emotional anxiety and apprehension about her future. As she put it, "It [back pain] was ruining my life. I couldn't work all day, I couldn't do the activities I enjoyed, and I couldn't try to have children."

Surgery alone often alleviates the physical symptoms, but most times it does not correct the underlying cause. Why did the disc herniate? When Helen asked her doctor this question, he shrugged his shoulders and said, "It just happens." Looking at the MRI and the sharp curve in the lumbar spine (lower back) where the disc herniated, Helen could see the problem.

Following surgery, Helen still had an increased risk of another episode of pain and injury in the same area of her body—lower back—if nothing was done to address the reason her disc initially herniated. To reduce this risk, Helen realized she needed to correct the underlying structural misalignment in her spine following surgery. Depending on the operation alone would not bring her the long-term confidence in her back that she desired. Hence, to achieve a better outcome than the operation alone would provide, she continues to work on her postural alignment to prevent a future surgery. I only question surgery when someone has an operation to fix symptoms without also addressing the underlying problem to help avoid the possibility of another surgery or painful episode. As you will learn in this chapter, a cycle of disability can occur when one only treats symptoms.

Limitations of Modern Medicine

Modern medicine is symptom-oriented, focused on ridding you of pain. Practitioners, from doctors to nurses to therapists, are limited not only in their scope of practice, but also in the time they can spend with patients. Additionally, they are restricted in the number of therapy treatments allowed by the insurance companies. These dedicated healthcare providers can only do so much within the confines of the medical system, and they really are trying their best to help patients. Unfortunately, many of us athletes continue to suffer, so we are still left searching for answers after the standard treatments have failed us.

Not knowing why you hurt is the hardest place to be during the healing process. It is a place of uncertainty about how to move forward, and you worry that activity might make things worse. If this is your situation, you have a choice to make about what to do next. Within the medical system, your options might include more diagnostic tests, different or stronger medications, increased physical therapy, injections, or surgery. Any of these treatments may absolutely be the correct path for you to take. Recall my tip from Chapter 4: If the medical intervention feels right—go for it. However, if you're not excited about your current options and want to try a different path, keep reading. We are going to dig deeper into your injury and the source of your pain.

Why You Hurt

Some critical questions we frequently forget to ask are, "*Why* did this injury happen?" or, "*Why* did this pain start?" For me, standard medical treatment left me wondering, "*Why did my left knee become damaged, but not my right? Why, after my knee surgeries, did I then have a hip problem, and why won't my back pain go away?*" We look to our diagnosis for answers, and it may seem obvious. You might have been diagnosed with a chronic condition (piriformis syndrome, shin splints, tennis elbow . . .) or you might have been told you have suffered a physical injury (torn cartilage, bulging discs, muscle strain . . .). This is why you hurt, and that is true. Each of these conditions and injuries is painful and represents damage that needs to be healed. However, for me as a coach, I want to go deeper. I want to know why these problems developed in the first place.

Chronic pain is different from an acute injury. For example, an acute injury like a broken bone is commonly fixed with a relatively straightforward procedure: surgery, if needed, to set the bones, followed by immobilization of the joint. Chronic pain, on the other hand, tends to come on gradually, slowly becoming worse, until the discomfort is too great to continue playing. You have a label for the pain—your diagnosis—but is that really the cause of your pain, or is it just a symptom? You might recall reading in Chapter 4 about my shock when I was told that the osteoarthritis in my hip was a symptom of joint misalignment.

It may be that you were predisposed to suffer this injury, like I was, because of my poor alignment and body mechanics. Putting all the answers together to your *why* questions will create a picture of the underlying dysfunction in your body. I asked myself:

Why can't I contract my left gluteal muscles?
Why is my right side always tighter than my left?
Why can I run without pain but cycling hurts?
Why is my right hip higher than my left?
Why can I balance better on my left foot?

Not asking *why* to discover the root cause of your pain can lead to a cycle of chasing symptoms. It starts with one joint, and spreads to another, and then another. For example, knee surgery, then a hip replacement, then a back procedure—that's the path I was going down.

I saw this same cycle—pain moving from joint to joint and spreading throughout the body—while working with ergonomic cases. I would be called in for an office workstation evaluation when an employee was complaining of wrist pain. Upon meeting with the employee, I'd ask about her wrist pain. In answer to this question, I routinely uncovered a history of symptoms. Now the pain was in the wrist, but previously it had been in the elbow or shoulder, on the same arm. Back pain was also common in these cases. Failing to ask *why* and to address the underlying cause of the pain, instead of just treating symptoms with ergonomic devices, prolonged the employee's suffering, as she chased symptoms around her body.

You have probably heard stories of people who have had multiple joints replaced or repeated back surgeries. Chronic pain and joint degeneration is caused by stress within the body. If the cause of this stress is not addressed, the unbalanced forces will just be redirected to other joints and soft tissues.[1] Thus, the body continues to break down and never fully heals. This will lead to an unending cycle of symptoms and invasive procedures. This cycle can be broken by correcting the underlying cause of the stress on your tissues and joints.

mind

Body-Wide Connections

To uncover the *why* underlying your pain, you need to understand how the body actually works, which might differ from what you learned in anatomy class. In school, I was taught that muscles are levers and pulleys, and that they work in isolation from the rest of the body. Muscles attach to two points, generally two bones, and they work in opposing pairs. When muscles are stimulated, they shorten, while the opposing muscles lengthen to produce movement. I learned that when muscles pull on bones, movement happens,[2] as shown in Figure 5-1.

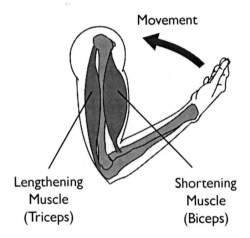

Although there is truth in the levers and pulleys model, this is a simplified view of the body. In reality, moving the arm has body-wide impacts, as Tom Myers, internationally known expert in fascia and author of

Figure 5-1. When your biceps muscles shorten, and triceps muscles lengthen, the lower arm moves up.[2]

Anatomy Trains®, discovered through his research. He found that nothing within the body moves in isolation. Muscles, bones and connective tissues are all intertwined, interdependent—they cannot be separated. Through careful dissections, Myers has documented these interconnected channels

93

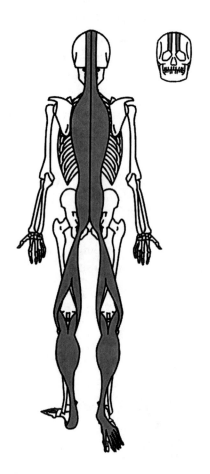

within the myofascial system of the body, which contain both the muscle (myo) and connective tissue (fascia). These linked lines of tissue, called the Anatomy Trains®, connect the body from head to toe. Movement in one part of the line, such as at the biceps, will have a corresponding effect up and down the myofascial line (Anatomy Train®). Likewise, a disruption in the myofascial line, such as tightness, reduced range of motion or impaired function, can cause compensation and pain in another part of the line or body.[3]

Take, for example, the Superficial Back Line, as shown in Figure 5-2, which runs from the bottom of the foot, up the back of the leg through the calves and hamstrings, to the pelvis and up the back muscles (erector spinae), and all the way over the head to the level of the eye brows. A restriction in any area of this line could cause problems anywhere along the Anatomy Train® from the bottom of the foot to the head and neck.[3] For instance, tightness in the calf could be related to back pain, or a headache could correspond to a problem in the hamstrings.

Figure 5-2. The Superficial Back Line is one of the Anatomy Trains® identified by Tom Myers.

Unfortunately, this concept of the body working together as an integrated whole is not how we typically think about the body. If you have been to the *Body Worlds Exhibition,*[4] which displays dissected human bodies in sports postures, you might have noticed how all of the connective tissue had been removed from the models to expose just the muscles and bones. This type of demonstration further sustains our segmented view of how the muscles and joints work independently from one another, which is not the case at all. The connective tissues link the body together in an interrelated web.[3]

How Your Body Distributes Strain

In addition to body-wide connections through the fascia, Myers' concept of an Anatomy Train® depends on viewing the body as a tensegrity structure. As I learned in his *Fascia and Movement Webinar Series,*

"Fascia + Tensegrity = The Anatomy of Connection."[5]

Before I define the characteristics of a tensegrity structure, let's talk about a simpler and more familiar structural design, such as that seen in a three-story building, as shown in Figure 5-3. A multi-story building is constructed by placing one floor on top of another. As the building grows taller, the downward compressive force through the structure increases.

Compression force is one way to support an object.[3] Your tendency, like mine was, might be to think of the body as a compressive structure in which the bones are stacked one on top of the other. The head sits on the neck, which is pushing down on the spine, pelvis, knees, etc. If you think of the body this way, there would be large compressive forces down at your feet. This traditional model of human structure assumes continuous compressive forces down the body.

The second force to consider in biological structures is tension. Objects can also be supported by tension,[3] as shown in Figure 5-4.

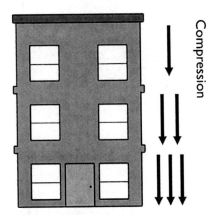

Figure 5-3. The compressive force in the first floor, which is supporting the two floors above, is much greater than in the top floor.

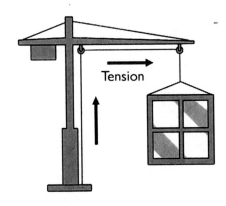

Figure 5-4. The crane supports a window at the end of a cable through tension in the wire.

95

A tensegrity structure combines the forces of compression and tension.[3] Figure 5-5(a) shows the design of a balanced tensegrity structure. In this model, Myers compares the dowel rods to bones and the elastic lines between them to the myofascia. The dowels (bones) provide the compressive force, which is pushing outward on the structure to maintain its shape. The elastics (myofascia) provide the tensional force, which is pulling inward. When these forces are balanced, the structure is stable, as shown in Figure 5-5(a).[3] As Myers explains it, "the dowels, the bones of this structure [...] are floating in space and they are held in space by the balance of the elastics, the muscles and the fascia, the myofascia. [...] The bones float inside the soft tissue."[6] Hence, the position of the bones is directed by the tension within the surrounding myofascia. Figure 5-6 is a representation of the human body as a tensegrity structure.

When an external force is placed on a tensegrity structure, shown in Figure 5-5(b), the strain is distributed through the elastics (myofascia) to the entire structure.[3] For example, if you fall on your right hip, the impact is going to spread throughout your body along your myofascia (elastics) and the Anatomy Trains®. The jolt of the fall is not going to just affect the hip; your whole body absorbs and distributes the forces generated with the fall. Changes

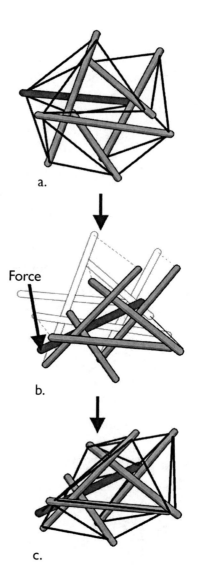

a.

Force

b.

c.

Figure 5-5. In a tensegrity structure the dowels are suspended by the elastics. Image (a) is an aligned structure. Image (b) is experiencing an external force in one area, which results in a deformation of the entire structure, Image (c).

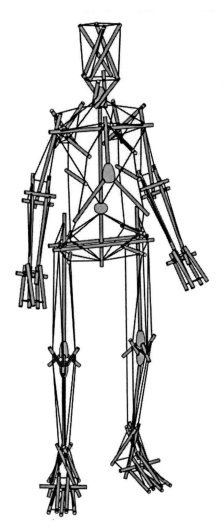

in tension in these soft tissues (elastics) at the hip and beyond could then alter the orientation of your bones (dowels) throughout your structure, as shown in Figure 5-5(c). When bones become misaligned due to soft tissue imbalances, movement patterns can be compromised, leading to pain and injury.

It is because of this body-wide response throughout the structure to an external force that a trauma in one area of the body can manifest as pain or injury in another location. In Myers' words, "The injury happens where it does because of inherent weakness or previous injury, not purely and always because of local strain."[3] In the example of falling on your hip, your right hip is the point of local strain, but injury and pain may be felt in another area of the body, one that was previously hurt or had weakness, such as the left shoulder. It is important to realize that the external force that alters the tension in the soft tissues does not have to be as dramatic as a fall. Also, it can take a long time for the injury or pain to develop from a slight alteration in the balance of your design. A minor bump of your leg on an object can create lasting tightness in the myofascia, which then creates pain months later. This is why you want to be vigilant about listening to the messages of your body and watching for changes in your posture. You will read more about this in Chapter 7.

Figure 5-6. The design of the human body combines compression through the bones and tension through the myofascia to maintain its form.

Kinetic Chains, Mobility and Stability

Remember the song "Dem Bones?" "Knee bone's connected to the thigh bone. Thigh bone's connected to the hip bone. Hip bone's connected to the back bone."[7] The bones throughout the body are connected through the soft tissues of the Anatomy Trains®. The position and movement of each bone affects the next; nothing works in isolation. This is referred to as the kinetic chain of the body.[8] This interconnection between everything in the body, not just the bones, explains why unhealthy changes happening in one part of the body can modify the mechanics of another part of the body and can create symptoms such as pain. Pete Egoscue likes to say that the body works as a "closely integrated unit."[1] Consequently, the movement or lack of motion in one joint influences the joints above and below it. Each joint is a separate link in the body's kinetic chain.

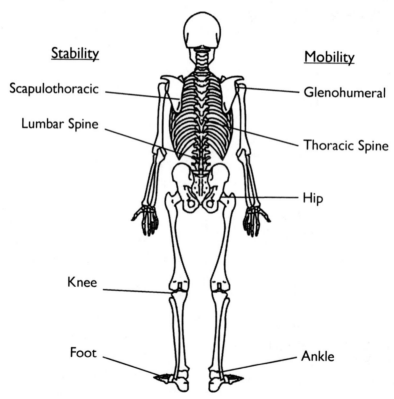

Figure 5-7. The joints in the body alternate between dominance in mobility or stability.

Your joints are designed to be both mobile and stable. Each of your joints is dominant in one of these abilities. The qualities of stability and mobility alternate, moving up toward the head,[8] as shown in Figure 5-7. Joint mobility is defined by Fabio Comana, faculty instructor at San Diego State University (SDSU) and National Academy of Sports Medicine (NASM), exercise physiologist, and speaker, as "the range of uninhibited movement around a joint or body segment."[8] Joint stability, on the other hand, is the "ability to maintain or control joint movement or position."[8] To paraphrase, you need to have sufficient range of motion (mobility) in your joint without it dislocating (stability). A deficiency in the mobility or stability of a joint can impact the surrounding joints, causing pain and injury.

If you ride a bike, you know what it feels like when you have a stiff link in your bike chain. With each revolution, there is a noticeable catch in the circle where pedaling becomes rough as the rigid section goes through the drivetrain. Each time the solid piece of chain passes through the cogs, the links on either side bend more to keep the wheels spinning. The same thing happens within the body. If one joint has become inflexible, the joints on either side of it move more to make up for the first joint's lost range of motion. When these compensating joints increase their mobility, they consequently give up some of their own stability. Thus, you have an inflexible joint surrounded by overly mobile and unstable joints. Ideally, this would never happen—a joint would not give up stability for mobility—but it is a common cause of injury and pain. This was the case for my client, Tarik.

A devoted cyclist, runner and cross-country skier, Tarik struggled with chronically tight hips, left knee pain with running (that turned to hip pain when he ran longer miles), and lower back pain when he classic cross-country skied. Although Tarik rode his bike nearly everywhere—he rarely used his car—he also rarely stretched his body. I suspected the cause of his pains might have been stemming from his hip tightness. His hips themselves, being directly located between his main sites of pain—the knees and the lower back—hurt on occasion. It's important to note here that the hips are designed to be the second most mobile joint in the body (with the shoulders being the most mobile joint). The knees and lower back are both stability joints with limited ranges of motion. In cases where the hips are restricted in movement, these surrounding stability joints will be forced to take on a larger mobility role to compensate. The stability joints—knees and lower back—will be forced to move in ways for which they are not designed. This additional movement can direct harmful forces through the joints, causing pain and injury.[8] This is what was happening to Tarik.

Upon testing Tarik's hip mobility, it was clear that his hips were locked up; they had very limited ability to move freely. He started an intensive daily program of hip-opening exercises along with techniques to maintain or improve his mobility and stability throughout his entire kinetic chain. Our fear was if the joints on the other sides of his painful ones lost their function, his pain might persist or become worse, or he could develop new symptoms. Happily, within a month of starting his program, Tarik's lower back was feeling better. Because he consistently followed his program and gained greater hip mobility, his pains continued to diminish, and his sports performance improved.

Tarik's pain was a result of limited mobility. Injuries can also arise when there is excessive mobility within muscles, joints and ligaments.

For example, as a former gymnast, I was accustomed to performing very deep stretching, to the point of being damaging to my body. With my fellow gymnasts, I would put my legs up between chairs in a split position to gain hyper-flexibility through the back of my legs, hips and pelvis. When forcing myself into this position, my body needed to gain increased length somewhere, and my muscles could only stretch so far. To gain this kind of hyper-mobility in the lower body, other structures are compromised, specifically the stability ligaments around the pelvis and hips. These ligaments are designed to hold the pelvis in a neutral position and the hips in alignment with the pelvis. Ligaments are strong bands, or sheets, of connective tissue that join bones. These tissues are not very pliable. Over-lengthening through excessive stretching (like I was doing) can lead to pelvic misalignments and instability in the hip joint.[9]

As I stretched, these ligaments became looser and longer, increasing the ability of my hips to slightly dislocate so I could gain deeper flexibility. My hips didn't actually come completely out of the socket, but they did move within the pelvis and changed orientation to accommodate greater mobility in a split position. My hips gave up stability for unhealthy mobility. Could this have been a precursor to my knee and hip injuries? You're nodding your head yes, and you're right. More about this in Chapter 6.

Treat the Cause of Your Pain and Injury, Not Your Symptoms

If you have pain in your feet and have been diagnosed with plantar fasciitis, it is natural to assume the problem is in your feet, right? Hopefully, you are starting to question this statement. This, however, is what my client Marilyn naturally thought:

> As an avid hiker, I became very discouraged when I ended up with a SEVERE case of plantar fasciitis in both feet! I tried many treatments for my pain: two podiatrists, 4 or 5 eight-week physical therapy sessions, foot vibrator, icing my feet, not hiking for TWO years, rolling my feet on a frozen bottle of water, acupuncture, and many more methods. Nothing seemed to relieve my pain.

By the time Marilyn entered my office, she was at the end of her rope and desperate for healing, as many of my clients are. Upon evaluation, I found Marilyn's pelvis to be twisted and tipped forward. Watching her walk, I noticed faulty gait mechanics with a lack of flexion and extension in her hips, and feet that turned out and rolled sideways. I concluded that her pelvic misalignment and compromised walking pattern were likely contributing to her pain. Upon discussing my findings with her, she mentioned noticing stiffness and discomfort in her hips. Additionally, she realized she had more trouble with her left hip, which was the same side as her more severe plantar fasciitis symptoms. This was an eye-opener for her, so she agreed to try a different approach to heal her pain. Before she saw me, Marilyn's therapy had all been directed from the knee down. She had done lots of calf stretching, tried various foot orthotics, and performed many types of the previously-mentioned foot manipulations (icing, rolling, acupuncture) with no long-term benefit.

For Marilyn to heal, her body needed to be treated as a connected whole from her head to her feet. I provided her with exercises directed to improve her hip function, pelvis position, and upper body postural deviations.

While doing an exercise to mobilize her hips, Marilyn noticed something that surprised her: "As I moved my hips through a range of motion, I was surprised to feel pain in my feet. Perhaps my hips are an issue that needs to be addressed for my feet to heal?" This experience cemented the connection between her hips and plantar fasciitis for her, so she diligently did her daily exercises. "After two and a half years of pain, Jessica found the magical exercise regimen for me! When I do the Egoscue® exercises, my feet do not hurt! What a relief!!!"

In addition to addressing Marilyn's pain through exercises for her lower body kinetic chain—foot to hip—I also gave her exercises for her upper body misalignments. I addressed her elevated left shoulder, left forward spine rotation, forward head posture, rounded shoulders and extended rib cage. Repositioning the upper body has an impact on how the forces are directed through the body down to the feet. Just try standing barefoot on a hard surface with your hands behind your head, which repositions your upper body, and notice how it changes the weight distribution in your feet as compared to having your hands by your sides. Note that if you are already well aligned in your upper body, any changes in weight distribution will be small and hard to detect.

Instead of treating the symptom—the pain in Marilyn's feet—I looked at her body as an integrated unit to find the driving cause of her pain. Myers has a saying regarding pain in the body: "The victim screams, while the criminal is silent."[5] Marilyn's feet were screaming, and quite loudly, while her hips were only whispering faintly; her crooked pelvis and unbalanced upper body were not making a sound. Marilyn's initial approaches to recovery were focused on treating her symptoms, but the underlying cause was ignored. Therefore, her pain relief was short lived.

Within our current medical system, our symptom-based approach to healing, it may be hard to accept that the cause of chronic pain is often located somewhere else in the body, some place that does not actually hurt. Generally, we associate the location of the pain with the cause of the pain. The medical community reinforces this "the problem is where the pain is" mentality. If you have foot pain, that is usually what is treated, while other contributing body asymmetries, dysfunctions and compensations are neglected. You may be feeling pain in your foot, but the forces creating that strain quite likely originate somewhere else. Given that your pain and the underlying problem are not always co-located, it should not be surprising when therapy focused on curing "where it hurts" does not work.

The manner in which Marilyn's foot was contacting the ground, and the forces her plantar fascia experienced while she hiked, were due to faulty body alignment and movement patterns above the foot. It was not until these unbalanced relationships and poor leg biomechanics were addressed that the strain on the tissues in her feet could be reduced and healed.

mind

A Note About Foam Rolling

Myers' book *Anatomy Trains®* has led to a proliferation of equipment for self-myofascial release, the most popular being the foam roller and various balls of different size and density. I have often recommended self-myofascial release to my clients to reduce muscle stiffness, break up adhesions (areas where soft tissues stick together), clear trigger points (tender spots), increase circulation, and improve range of motion. I find it particularly useful before doing corrective posture exercises and after a workout. When used in this way, I fully support the practice.

My issue with foam rolling and the like is when it is used as a crutch to keep playing despite an obvious imbalance. When used in this manner, self-myofascial release is doing no more than treating a symptom without addressing the underlying cause. There is a reason you have recurring one-sided body tightness. Just rolling it away is avoiding the issue and going to perpetuate the problem, which may become worse and spread.

I mention this because I did it. This is how I dealt with the ache in my right hip during cross-country ski season. I would develop unrelenting tightness in the hip when skate skiing. It was not pain per se, but it was very restricted, immobile tissue. I used my foam roller, tennis balls and softballs to ease the incessant knot before and after my time on skis. Of course, as soon as I would go back out on the snow and skate, my hip tightness would return, quicker and quicker each time. I have memories of many skate races where I was in agony. I still raced—yet I became happier each year as early February and the local skate marathon passed so I could put those skis aside and only classic ski.

Although I was trying to address the underlying issue at the time, my efforts weren't successful. I was still in the mindset of ignoring and pushing through my pain. *Such a hard habit to break!* Now I can skate ski without discomfort and don't use the foam roller as a crutch. I'm concerned, though, about how many people are using foam rolling as a Band-Aid and are continuing to play through injury and pain. I doubt I'm alone in abusing this technique.

Cautions About Joint Taping and Bracing

What happens when the kinetic chain is voluntarily altered through taping or bracing? It is common to see rows of athletes lining up in the training room before any athletic practice or competition and having various body parts taped so they can go play. I did it.

Every day before gymnastics practice in college, I, along with many of my teammates, would stop at the training center and take my seat on the table to have my left ankle taped. As an athlete, you don't think much about it, except that you need to get to practice early to be ready on time. What was wrong with my ankle? I didn't have any idea. Was I doing any therapy on my ankle to recover so I wouldn't have to tape it? Absolutely not. And I didn't care. I just wanted to go to practice and prepare for competition. This is a typical athletic mindset about injuries: ignore and push through. The ankle pain was merely an inconvenience that was getting in my way of doing what I wanted. I didn't care about healing my ankle. I was simply interested in a way to mask its pain so I could keep playing. Taping provided relief; it made the problem go away, so I did it. In my athletic community, taping was not only accepted, it was expected. It was a normal part of the game. The common philosophy of my coaches, trainers and teammates was that the body is weak and must be braced from the outside. It needs external support to compensate for a lack of internal stability. We believed that gymnastics was hard on the body, so extra joint support was required to sustain the demands of the sport.

Taping is a stopgap measure to allow the game to go on. When taped, my ankle lacked its natural function and range of motion. The demands of my sport did not decrease, though. I continued to ask my body to do the same amount of work, at the same intensity, without full use of my ankle. As noted in Figure 5-7, the ankle is primarily a mobility joint. By tightly taping it in a fixed position, essentially making it a non-flexible stability joint, I set myself up for joint problems: long-term muscular compensations that would over-stress the joints and tissues above and below the ankle as well as do continual damage to the ankle itself. Let me explain: My ankle could not do the work required to perform the demanding gymnastics routines. I still had to attain the same dramatic positions, even if my foot could not bend. Since the restrictive taping had taken away the ankle's mobility, the surrounding joints and tissues had to create additional movement. The knee, being the closest joint to the ankle, was the first to come to my assistance. It provided the needed mobility beyond its normal capabilities so that I could perform. In doing so, the knee sacrificed its stability to the point of the joint becoming injured. Recall that this should not happen—joints giving up stability for mobility—and often leads to breakdown.

Is it a coincidence that all four of my joint surgeries—three knee surgeries and one hip surgery—have been on my left side, leading directly up from my injured ankle? I think not. The inappropriate movement patterns that began with my taped ankle in gymnastics were never rehabilitated. The pain eventually went away, but the flawed movements the body had learned while the ankle was taped lived on. For many years, even decades after my gymnastics career, my left ankle popped and cracked when I walked, and my whole left leg felt disconnected, functioning separately from my right. It seemed as if I had two different legs at times. They were not coordinated, and sometimes moving was painful. All this so I could continue to compete in college gymnastics. Oh, the choices I made . . . If only I had known the consequences!

As I learned, restricting the motion in a joint is not a good long-term solution to pain. It actually creates more, increasingly severe injuries beyond the initial joint. Perpetual joint taping weakens the joint, which furthers the imbalance and prolongs the recovery. Dependence on external bracing sets athletes up for future pain and disability. Taping will help athletes return to the field, court or trail, but it should only be used short-term while the injury is healing. Also, it should be done in conjunction with rehabilitation to regain internal joint stability so that the athlete does not become dependent on taping. Rehabilitation should include re-learning proper movement patterns to reduce the chance of either repeating the injury or hurting another part of the body.

Joint taping not only causes physical damage but also impacts the athlete's psyche. This is one of the scenarios in which sports teaches us to ignore pain and dissociate from the sensations in our body, which was discussed in Chapter 2. We override the protective signal the body is sending so we can continue to play. This mental habit, developed during the formative athletic years regarding pain and injuries, can be hard to break and can last a lifetime. As we age, we may no longer tape our joints, even though Kinesio Tape is quite popular. Instead, we might graduate to store-bought or prescription braces, pain-relieving medications, numbing injections, surgery and joint replacements—all the while perpetuating and reinforcing the cycle of compensation, imbalance, and pain.

Choosing Your Treatment Path

How are you going to treat your injury? Will you choose a quick fix that addresses symptoms? Or will you take a more integrated approach, looking at your whole body, asking *why*, and treating the cause of your pain? Initially, I just treated my symptoms where it hurt. I didn't know any better, and, as with all decisions in life, made the best choice I could with the information I had at the time. I hope I have given you some information that is challenging your thinking about how you are going to approach your healing. I also hope that I have pushed you to look past your symptoms, to gain a deeper understanding about your body and the interaction of all of your systems. After all, this is a book about holistic healing. Before you choose your next step, let me tell you a little more about my journey and why I chose posture therapy to treat my pain. The next chapter exposes the start of my healing journey—the good, the bad, and the posturally ugly.

mind

Summary

How you treat your injury will be influenced by your mindset, shaped by your previous experiences, beliefs and environment. Following the standard medical approach to healing can be highly effective, or it can leave you in pain with a reduced ability to play sports. To gain full recovery to the level you desire, you might have to go outside the medical model and take a more holistic approach. Instead of treating your superficial symptoms, you will need to go deeper, asking *why* the injury occurred, and correct the underlying cause of your pain.

The cause of your injury is often not located in the same place as your pain because strain, such as that caused by a fall, is distributed throughout your structure. The body is intricately connected from head to toe in a kinetic chain of soft tissues and bones. Strain in one area of the body is transmitted via compression and tension forces along these integrated myofascial lines, called Anatomy Trains®. Pain and injury often occurs at the site of weakness along these lines, which is frequently different from the local area of trauma. Hence, treatment is needed in a place of the body outside the location of pain.

Joints are designed to be both mobile and stable, but they are dominant in one or the other. Injuries can occur when joints are compromised in these abilities, particularly when stability joints are forced to take on excessive mobility. Foam rolling is a popular technique used to keep the muscles limber and joints healthy, but this practice can be abused. When a consistent pattern of muscle tightness is present, modalities beyond self-myofascial release with a foam roller are required for healing. Likewise, taping and bracing joints is not a long-term solution to treating an injury and should only be used in combination with rehabilitation of the injured body part.

Game Winning Strategies

1. Explore Your Healing Mindset

Your previous experiences, beliefs and environment influence the treatment path you will choose to treat your injury. Questions to consider:

What has worked in the past for you or others you know who've had the same or similar injury or pain?

What do you truly believe your body needs to heal?

What do the people around you—those who care about you, have a strong influence, and whose opinion you respect—advise for you?

2. Uncover *Why* You Hurt

Why you hurt may not be straightforward because your injury is a symptom, not the underlying cause, of your suffering. Make a list of all the *why* questions you have about your pain, injury and body. Write down everything you've noticed about any side-to-side differences. Consider asymmetries in mobility and stability, strength and function. Also notice patterns related to the kinetic chain, such as neighboring joints on the same side of the body being affected. Use the *Why* self-discovery questions listed earlier in this chapter as a guide and add any additional ones you have.

After you've made your list, re-read your questions and write down any answers, observations, trends or similarities that come to mind. Write down anything that seems to be related and could shed light on your situation.

Looking at this information, what thoughts do you have about the true cause of your pain or injury?

mind

Align Your Body

2

6

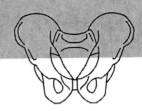

The Posture—Pain Connection

*A*fter four joint surgeries and numerous rounds of physical therapy, I was still in pain. Although valuable, adding chiropractic, massage, acupuncture and yoga to my healing remedies didn't bring long-term relief. This was not acceptable to me. I was too young, strong and fit to give up my athletic life. There had to be another option, and I was determined to find it.

After my third left knee surgery, I commented to my orthopedic surgeon that I felt like there was something beyond my knee that was causing it to degenerate. I didn't know what I was talking about; it was just a sense I had, so I was hoping my doctor could enlighten me. His answer was to do 300 leg lifts a day to build up my thigh (quadriceps) muscles, specifically my vastus medialis oblique (VMO). That didn't seem like a plausible solution to me, not only because of the ridiculous number, but more because I couldn't execute the exercise correctly. While in physical therapy, I worked on leg lifts, but it was clear my body couldn't find the right muscles to fire and strengthen while doing the exercise. Even pasting electrodes on my leg and zapping my muscles wasn't much use.

Following my hip surgery, I continued trying to ease my pain but wasn't getting anywhere. I was frustrated, confused and very upset. I didn't know what to do next or whom to ask for help. Fortunately, that was when my massage therapist, Susan, provided me with the answer to my intuitive sense—that there was a bigger cause for my body's continued decline. She told me about body alignment and re-introduced me to the Egoscue Method®.[1] She planted the seed that my posture was the larger issue I needed to address.

Living in a Crooked Body

On June 13, 2008, nearly a year following arthroscopic surgery to repair my left hip labral tear, I had my initial session with an Egoscue Method® therapist, John. The surgery had helped my hip pain, but it was still restricted and popping. I broke down in tears the first time my hip popped after surgery. I thought that would clear up with the operation. Naively, I had thought the surgery would fix everything, but I was wrong. I also continued to suffer debilitating lower back pain and extreme upper body tightness, and I had given up professional mountain biking. Prior to seeing John, I completed a detailed intake form listing all my previous surgeries, pains and lifestyle factors such as stress management, sleep and hydration. When I met with John, we talked at length about my injuries, and we discussed how posture and function might be playing a role in my pain. Part of the initial session included taking four posture pictures—front, back and both sides—to ensure consistency in my position. Here's my recollection of the experience:

I stood anxiously in front of the digital camera in my shorts and sports bra. John told me not to pose—to stand as I naturally would—and clicked off four mug-shot-like posture photos. He slowly circled around me, studying my joint alignment. I was sure he wouldn't find anything to fix. Boy, was I wrong! Fortunately, he was kind in his descriptions and didn't elaborate on his findings. Let's just say there were plenty of postural disparities to address. He developed my personalized daily menu of exercises (E-cises™), stretches, repositioning postures, and functional strengthening movements; I handed over my credit card, enrolling in the largest package of sessions he offered. It was a huge financial investment, but my body and athletic future were worth the commitment of funds, time and energy if this approach would provide the relief I needed and would allow me to get back on my bike.

Figure 6-1 shows my left side posture. Like many cyclists, my posture had become altered from the repetitive sitting and forward flexion on the bike. Not only was I sitting when I rode, but I also had a sedentary desk job. Since the body adapts to the positions frequently assumed, it can get stuck in its athletic postures. My body was pedaling a bike 24/7.

If your body consistently senses a postural misalignment, it accommodates to hold that position. The muscles and surrounding connective tissues (myofascia) modify their length and tension to alter the placement of the bones and resulting posture of your body. Consequent to these changes, my spine became overly curled. The spine has three distinct curves in the lower back (lumbar), mid-upper back (thoracic) and neck (cervical). Each of these areas of my spine was altered. My cervical spine was too straight and had lost its backward curve, while my thoracic spine was rounding excessively forward through my shoulders, similar to the position I was in when holding onto the handlebars of my bike, and my lumbar spine was arching dramatically backward. My distorted lower back curve counterbalanced the rounding in my thoracic spine. The rounded spinal posture of my mid-upper back continued into my neck, thrusting my head forward.

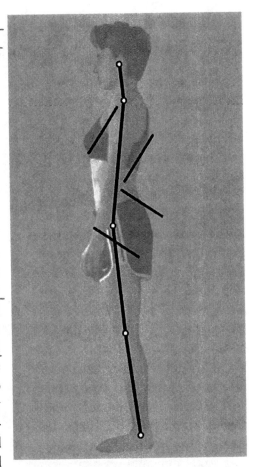

Figure 6-1. My side posture demonstrates exaggerated spinal curves: the line drawn down my side should be straight.

(Sometimes postural misalignments can be deceiving and hard to spot, as in this case. You might think I am actually extended in my thoracic spine, but that is an illusion created by the asymmetries in my lumbar spine and pelvis below.) To bring my eyes level to the horizon when standing, I overly lengthened the front of my torso and compressed my lower back. My chest was lifted up and rib cage flared out. This positioned my shoulders so far back that they were no longer aligned with my hips and pelvis, which was subsequently tilting too far forward. These deviations are shown by the lines parallel to each side of the rib cage and pelvis in Figure 6-1.

115

Although my front and back views were less dramatic, they still showed asymmetries. I always find it easier to see these differences from the back view—when we are less likely to be posing, as shown in Figure 6-2.

In my back posture, you'll notice a slightly higher left shoulder, a higher right hip, collapsing ankles, and an excessive lower back curve and tightness. You might also be able to see the additional space between the right side of my body and my right arm, along with a more defined curve on my right side between the top of my shorts and bottom of my bra. My right arm also hangs more forward than my left arm. Notice how you can see my left elbow clearly, while the right has less detail. How beautifully crooked I was. And I thought my posture was good! *Ha!*

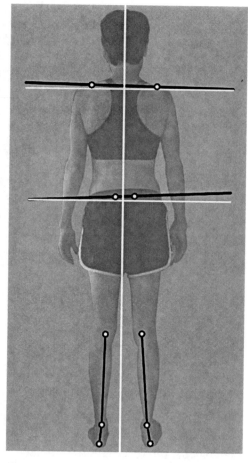

Figure 6-2. Many postural asymmetries can be seen in the back view of my posture; the main ones are highlighted.

Hip and Pelvis Asymmetries

One of my primary postural deviations was in my hips and pelvis. This is a common site of imbalance and pain for many people. It is also an initial area targeted for treatment, according to Pete Egoscue: "Eliminating hip dysfunction is one of our top priorities simply because of the hips' central role."[2]

I've heard Egoscue Method® therapists refer to the pelvis as the second brain of the body because of its central location and the dual roles it provides. First, the pelvis is where we move from. Movement is generated from the pelvis and hips together, transferring power to the limbs. Second, the pelvis provides the structural base of support for our upper body. If the pelvic foundation beneath is not solid, shifts can happen in the body above. Let's take a closer look at the posture of the pelvis and hips.

Anatomically, the pelvis links the spine to the hips and upper leg bones (Figure 6-3). The human pelvis, as shown in Figure 6-4, is comprised of not one, but three bones: the sacrum at the base of the spine and two hip bones on either side.[3]

The hip bone is divided into four sections: the ilium at the top, ischium in the back, and pubis in the front. The hip bone also contains a depression called the acetabulum (Figure 6-5).[3]

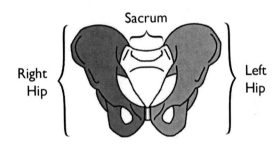

Figure 6-4. The three pelvic bones are the right and left hip bones and the sacrum.

Figure 6-5. The hip bone is divided into the ilium, ischium, pubis and acetabulum.

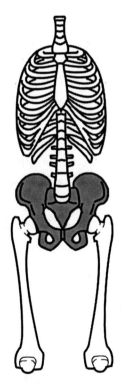

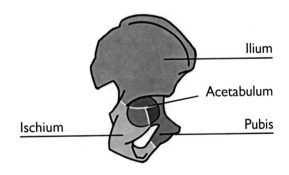

Figure 6-3. The pelvis connects the upper and lower body.

body

For simplicity, I am going to use the term "hip bone" in my discussion. The hip bones join into the sacrum on the back of the body, creating the sacroiliac joint (SIJ), and are held together with cartilage at the pubic symphysis in the front. This flexible design enables independent movement of the right and left sides of the pelvis (hip bones), which is essential for walking, as shown in Figure 6-6. If the pelvis were one solid bone, you wouldn't be able to walk. You could only hop, which doesn't require opposing flexion and extension of the hip bones.

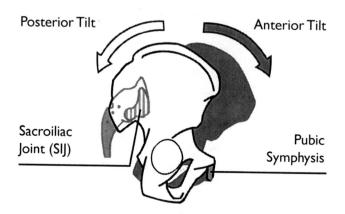

Posterior Tilt   Anterior Tilt

Sacroiliac Joint (SIJ)

Pubic Symphysis

Figure 6-6. The hip bones tilt in opposing directions when walking: one tilts forward (anterior) into flexion, while the other tilts backward (posterior) into extension.

Pelvic asymmetries can happen in three dimensions. (1) The hip bones can rotate around the spine, though the spine often follows the hip bones so that one side of the pelvis—right or left—is forward or behind the other side, Figure 6-7(a). (2) The hip bones can also raise or lower on either side so that one hip bone is above or below the other, Figure 6-7(b). (3) The hip bones can tilt too far forward (anterior) or backward (posterior) on one or both sides, Figure 6-7(c).[4]

My pelvis was skewed in all of these dimensions: my right hip bone was elevated and rotated forward compared to the left, and both sides of my pelvis—right and left hip bones—were tilted too far forward, more so on the right. If you think of the pelvis as a bowl filled with water, in a neutral position the pelvic bowl is slightly tilted forward and easily holds the water, Figure 6-8(a). My pelvis, however, was tipped sideways and rotated toward the left. It was tilted so far forward that any water in my pelvic bowl would be spilling out, with most the water cascading down the front of my left leg, Figure 6-8(b).

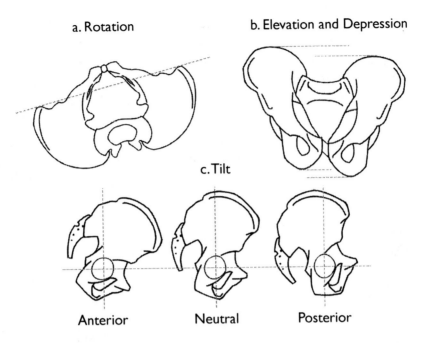

a. Rotation

b. Elevation and Depression

c. Tilt

Anterior   Neutral   Posterior

Figure 6-7. There are three asymmetries of the pelvis—(a) left and right rotation, (b) elevation and depression and (c) anterior and posterior tilt.

body

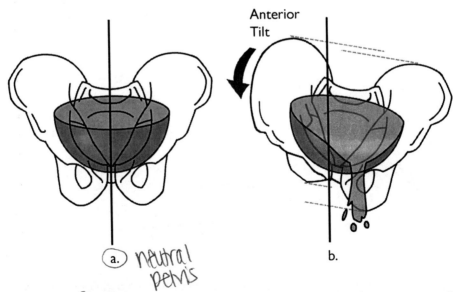

Anterior
Tilt

a. neutral pelvis

b.

Figure 6-8. (a) A neutral pelvis with a slight anterior tilt of both hip bones. (b) My tilted and rotated pelvis.

119

The hip joint is where the top of the leg bone (femur), in the shape of a ball, fits into the acetabulum in the hip bone of the pelvis, also known as the hip socket. The ball on the top of the femur is often referred to as the hip, as shown in Figure 6-9. Both the hip and acetabulum are lined with soft tissue (cartilage) to enable smooth joint mechanics. Your hip joint is a ball and socket joint, similar to the shallower glenohumeral joint at the shoulder, which is a partial ball and socket joint. Ball and socket joints can move in all directions. These ball and socket joints rely on muscles, ligaments and connective tissues to keep the bones positioned in the joint.[3]

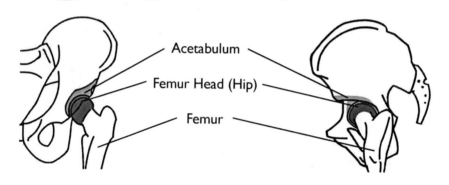

Figure 6-9. When the pelvis and hip joint are in a neutral orientation (healthy alignment), there is no contact between the hip and cartilage of the acetabulum.

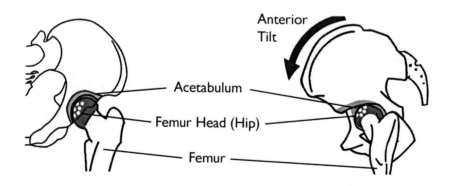

Figure 6-10. The pelvis has tilted forward. This puts the hip joint in an unhealthy alignment in which the hip is in contact with the cartilage of the acetabulum, causing breakdown, as indicated by the white spots.

If the pelvic bones are asymmetrical in any of the three dimensions, as shown in Figure 6-7—one hip bone rotated forward or backward of the other, one hip bone higher or lower than the other, or one hip bone tilted forward or backward of the other—the orientation of the hip within the acetabulum can become altered. In these skewed pelvic positions, the hip may migrate into a new location within the acetabulum, bumping up into the cartilage, as shown in Figure 6-10. In this orientation, the forces directed through the hip joint with movement will begin to wear the cartilage away.

It is at this time that your doctor tells you there is a hole in your hip joint, which is bone on bone, and you'll need a hip replacement . . . when you're in excruciating pain and thoroughly debilitated. Ah, how I remember those words well. But, you might be thinking, if the soft tissues—ligaments, muscles, fascia, etc.—are holding the hip and pelvis in a bad position, can't that be changed to allow the cartilage to regenerate? Yes, good question and observation! I'll discuss that when I talk about treatment. But now I want to talk about how the position of the hips affects the knees.

When the hip becomes misaligned, the knee joint, which is also held together by soft tissue and is at the other end of the femur bone, is also compromised. This is why Egoscue Method® therapists say that the knee is a window into the hip. For instance, if the femur is positioned pointing inward, the posture of the knee and hip joints are both affected. My femurs were both positioned inward, more so on the left side. So, it could be deduced that my hips were also pointed inward. To counter my hip and knee positions, my lower legs and feet pointed outward (like a duck), creating torsion at my knee joints, as shown in Figure 6-11.

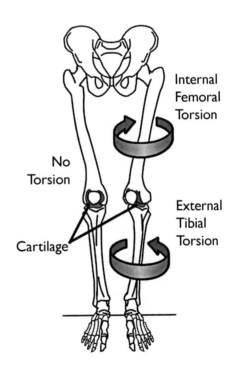

Internal Femoral Torsion

No Torsion

Cartilage

External Tibial Torsion

Figure 6-11. Knee torsion and cartilage (meniscus) damage happen when the upper and lower leg bones do not line up straight atop each other.

body

121

With misaligned bones at my knee joints, the fluid mechanics of bending and straightening my knees was impaired. Please notice the cartilage between the leg bones in Figure 6-11. Now imagine what happened to that soft tissue each time I took a step on my twisted knee. That poor cartilage, subjected to the uneven forces of the bones during movement, was being unevenly worn and eventually tore on my more twisted left side. A meniscus tear in the knee can be the symptom of postural misalignment and faulty motion.

The thing to take away from all of this is that asymmetries in the pelvis can show up as pain and injury both above and below this central joint. This is why the pelvis is a primary focus of posture correction. During my client posture assessments, I pay close attention to pelvic position. If asymmetries are found in the pelvis, that is where my coaching begins. (You'll read more about this in Chapter 9.) Many times, gaining equality in the pelvis relieves symptoms in other parts of the body, which are secondary to this fundamental misalignment.

Considerations for Leg Length Discrepancies

Clients often tell me their legs are different lengths. When they lay down on an examiner's table, one leg appears longer, and the practitioner informs them that their legs are different lengths. Or perhaps they have been told this by the tailor when having their pants hemmed. Some clients have been given lifts to put in their shoes to correct the imbalance. Early in my therapy, I was given such an insert. *It made my pain worse!* I quickly removed the offending piece of foam. Adding a lift to my shoe to reinforce my asymmetry never made sense to me. *Are my legs really different lengths? Should I be perpetuating this imbalance by placing a lift in my shoe? Wouldn't it be better to correct the discrepancy?*

It is rare for the leg bones to be uneven.[2] In my experience, leg length discrepancies without birth defects, leg breaks or surgery are NOT the result of different length bones, called "actual leg length"[5] discrepancies. Rather, what I see more commonly are "apparent leg length"[5] discrepancies, where the bones are the same length but *appear* shorter or longer because of muscle imbalances and asymmetries in the hips and pelvis.

As noted earlier, the pelvis can become out of alignment in three dimensions (Figure 6-7), which changes the hip's position within the pelvis and the orientation of the soft tissues. Hips can move within the socket—up, down, forward and backward. If the pelvis is asymmetrical and the hip position shifts in the socket, it could make the leg appear shorter or longer.[6] Review my posture in Figure 6-2. Viewing my elevated right hip bone, you might assume that my right leg is longer. If, however, my right hip were positioned farther down in the socket (healthy alignment), away from the acetabular cartilage, while the left was pushed up into the socket (unhealthy alignment), in contact with the acetabular cartilage—creating the hole—the leg bones could still be the same length, even though the right leg *appears* longer, and the left leg *appears* shorter. In this case, it might be helpful to view the left hip bone as depressed rather than the right hip bone as elevated. This pelvis and hip asymmetry can be perceived as a leg length discrepancy, as shown in Figure 6-12. Treating this unbalanced position with a lift was not going to fix the underlying problem: my hip and pelvis misalignments.

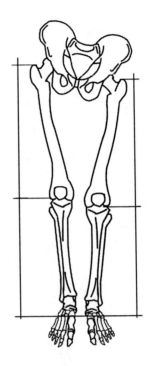

Figure 6-12. An asymmetrical pelvis can create the appearance of a leg length discrepancy when hip orientation within the socket changes.

body

Aligned Posture

We are designed to have our load-bearing joints—shoulders, hips, knees and ankles—positioned at 90-degree angles to each other from the front and side views, as shown in Figures 6-13 and 6-14. When in alignment, the left

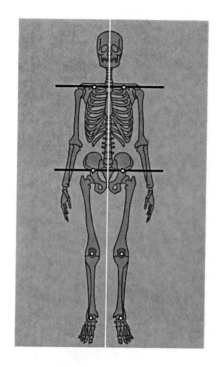
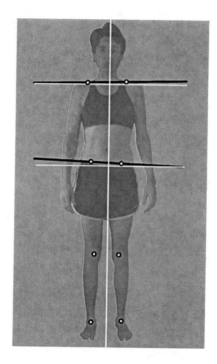

ideal posture

Figure 6-13. The image on the left is ideal front posture, in contrast to my posture on the right.

and right load-bearing joints should be horizontally level with each other and in a straight line vertically with the joints above and below. The knees and feet face straight ahead; the rib cage is centered in the torso above a level and neutral pelvis; the head is balanced evenly on top; weight is equally distributed through both feet; and the spine is in its natural curves without rotation or side bending.[2]

When your body is in the ideal posture, your muscles are balanced at their optimal length and tension, your joints are aligned, and you are strong. Regaining aligned posture, or at least getting closer to this ideal, is the goal of posture therapy and coaching. You don't have to attain perfect alignment to reduce your pain. The closer you get to the ideal, the better you'll feel and the lower your chance of injury.

Although injuries can happen when we are still, many more occur when we move. As I stated in the introduction, it is the *position and condition* of the body we bring into sports that matters. If we don't have good static postural alignment, we are more apt to hurt and to play poorly. Katy Bowman, a well-renowned movement biomechanist, explains why: "The reason we're

124

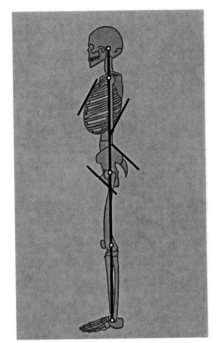
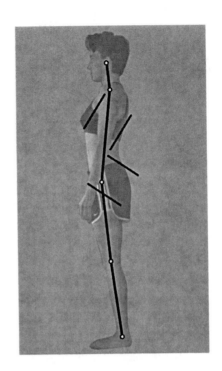

ideal left side posture

body

Figure 6-14. The image on the left is ideal left side posture, in contrast to my posture on the right.

even considering how your structure is oriented has to do with the forces that are created once you're moving."[7] So, the importance of static, aligned posture becomes critical when we move because of the forces generated. These forces are a result of loads. In a static postural assessment, I am looking at the position of the "load-bearing joints." How the load is transmitted through these joints determines if we suffer chronic pain and injury.

The Role of Loads and Forces in Chronic Pain and Injury

Bowman has a great discussion about loads in her book, *Move Your DNA*.[8] If you are into this sort of thing, definitely check it out. In her example, she demonstrates several ways to carry 13 pounds of pumpkin. Whether she is carrying one large pumpkin or several small pumpkins, the position in which she carries the fruit determines the load on her body. As she explains, the load is not the 13 pounds of pumpkin, but rather the act of carrying it and the forces that are created when she moves. Carrying the pumpkin on her head will create a different load through her load-bearing joints than holding multiple pumpkins in front of her body or balancing the pumpkins at her sides. As Bowman says:

> Every unique joint configuration, and the way that joint configuration is positioned relative to gravity, and every motion created, and the way that motion was initiated, creates a unique load that in turn creates a very specific pattern of strain in the body.[8]

When you are in aligned posture, the unrelenting, downward force of gravity is sent through your bones, making them stronger. Yes, good posture helps to prevent osteoporosis. However, when your body alignment deviates from this ideal, your muscles take on additional postural work, even before you move. You are no longer using your bones for support. The work of holding your body up is largely transferred to your muscles. Just looking at the image of my misaligned side view posture in Figure 6-14, you can imagine the additional stress that is being placed on my lower back and neck muscles just to maintain an upright position against gravity. My lower back and anterior (front) neck muscles are shortened, while the opposite is happening on the other side of the body—my posterior (back) neck and abdominal muscles are lengthened. These muscles can't relax when I'm upright, so they just become tighter, more immobile, and more painful.

Now take this distorted static posture into movement, and I'll have problems because of the forces generated through the joints as a response to the load of the activity. For instance, hiking creates a load on my joints as my body weight is carried through space. The hiking movements create forces that are transmitted throughout my body. When my hip and knee joints are not aligned correctly, these forces, including gravity, will be directed through the joints at awkward angles, causing increased strain, breakdown, and inflammation in the soft tissues (including the cartilage) that surround the joints.

In most sports, however, force is also coming from the ground up. This upward force is referred to as ground reaction force (GRF).[9] GRF counters gravity and body weight, as shown in Figure 6-15. For example, when we hit the ground while running, which is an integral part of many sports—soccer, field hockey, basketball, ultimate Frisbee, triathlon and more—the ground hits us back, as explained by Newton's Third Law of Motion: "For every action there is an equal and opposite reaction."[9] If this upward GRF encounters a postural deviation or "weak link" in the body, such as a knee or hip that is rotated inward or a back that is overly arched, pain and injury can develop in this area of the body.[10]

Recall that my left hip was locked into a skewed angle within my pelvis without any space between the acetabular cartilage. The loads of my activities, combined with my postural deviations, created excess force within my hip joint.

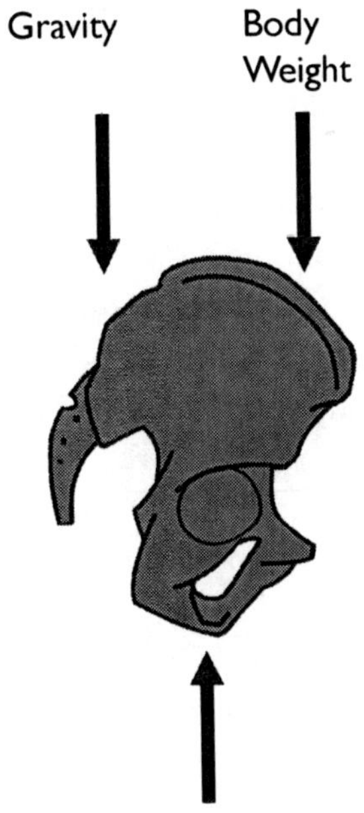

When the bones are not in proper position, stress and friction develop within a joint, which wears away and tears the delicate soft tissues. I was told I had a hole in the cartilage surrounding my hip joint. The misaligned bones had worn through the cartilage in one spot. Another way to view this is as follows: If you take your fist and put it in the palm of your opposite hand, and you continually rub the same spot, eventually the skin will turn red, then bleed, and so on. To fix the problem, you'd stop rubbing the same spot, which is essentially what you are doing by correcting misaligned posture. More to come on this in Chapter 8. This is an example of "wear and tear" injuries (mentioned in the introduction) being the result of microtraumas that are caused by misaligned posture and poor body mechanics.

Now that you've seen my posture and have learned how position affects pain, it's your turn. In the next chapter, you'll be analyzing your own posture and considering if your alignment might be contributing to your current injury, pain, or discomfort.

Gravity   Body Weight

Ground Reaction

Figure 6-15. The forces present during movement—gravity and ground reaction—in combination with body weight can cause damage when joints are misaligned.

body

Summary

Chronic pain is often connected to faulty posture. Misaligned (faulty) posture was the reason for my injuries and pain; it was the underlying cause of my suffering; and it explained why I was not improving with traditional or complementary medical approaches. An unbalanced skeleton reveals weakness, whereas joint alignment expresses strength. Ideal posture has the load-bearing joints—shoulders, hips, knees and ankles—horizontally and vertically aligned with each other.

The pelvis is the foundation of aligned posture. It consists of three bones—right and left hip bones and sacrum. The pelvis provides the foundational support for the upper body and is also where many movements originate in coordination with the hip. This central structure connects the upper and lower body. It can become asymmetrical in three ways—rotation, elevation/depression, and tilt disparities. If the pelvis is out of balance, repercussions can be felt throughout the body. Improper alignment of the hip within the acetabulum of the pelvis can cause cartilage degeneration, apparent leg length discrepancies, altered movement mechanics and pain. Knee position is commonly compromised when hip and pelvis postures are deviated, thus increasing the risk of pain and injury in this joint.

When a load is applied to a crooked body through movement, the forces that are generated can be misdirected into the soft tissues and joints, causing breakdown, pain, and inflammation. *That's why posture matters!* When joints are aligned, forces are distributed evenly through the body's structure without damage.

Game Winning Strategies

1. Learn More

Accepting that posture was the cause of my pain and injuries and committing to this treatment path required that I gain abundant knowledge about the posture-pain connection. Here are a few websites to check out for more information.

The Pain Free Athlete Blog
www.thepfathlete.com/blog

The Egoscue Method®
www.egoscue.com

Postural Restoration Institute®
www.posturalrestoration.com

2. Analyze Yourself

Please plan adequate time for the next chapter. It is interactive, and it is all about you. You will explore your alignment and become more aware of your body position, habits that may be molding your posture, and movement patterns.

body

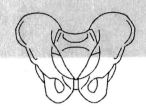

Examining Your Posture

*H*urrah! This chapter is all about you. In the previous chapter, I used myself as a postural example. Now it's time to take a look at you. From what you have read so far, do you think posture could be an underlying cause of your chronic pain or increased susceptibility to injury? I understand if you are not convinced that there is anything wrong with your posture. It took me a long time to make the connection and commit to changing my alignment. In my experience, however, many chronic soft tissue injuries and pain that haven't responded to traditional methods come down to postural misalignments and faulty movement patterns.

In this chapter, you'll be doing a self-assessment using principles taught by Egoscue University®.[1] In the assessment you'll be analyzing your posture, checking out your shoes, observing the weight distribution in your feet, and answering several questions about your body. By the end you'll have a clearer picture of yourself. Let's start by looking at your body and how your load-bearing joints—shoulders, hips, knees and ankles—line up.

Additional copies of the self-assessment tools—stick figure models, foot outlines, motion self-assessment charts—are available for download on my website: www.thepfathlete.com/resources.

Posture Self-Assessment

Please take a moment to do these self-tests before moving on to the next section. This assessment is just for you, though it might be helpful and more fun to do with a friend or partner. It will give you insight into your body and provide a baseline for your position. No one is perfect. And, the good news is that you can change your posture, but you need to know the starting point. Be brave! Let's begin.

Front View Analysis

When looking at your body from the front, you are measuring your side-to-side balance. You are noticing the symmetry, or lack of symmetry, in the right and left halves of your body. Ideally, if you dropped a plumb line down the center of your body, it would evenly separate your body into symmetrical right and left halves.

Step 1. Position Yourself

Stand facing forward in front of a full-length mirror in a relaxed position, wearing minimal clothing and no shoes.

Step 2. Observe Your Posture

What follows are several questions, starting with your feet and working up the body, to direct your self-assessment. There are numerous hints and notes to help you determine your responses. Record your answers in the space below each question or in your journal.

Do both feet face straight ahead?

Is one foot positioned ahead of the other? Which one is forward? (Note: A forward foot generally indicates a rotation of the body in that direction.)

Is one hand positioned ahead of the other? Which one is forward? (Note: This indicates rotation in the mid-upper back [thoracic spine].)

Is one side of your pelvis positioned more forward than the other? (Hint: Place your hands on the fronts of both sides of your hip bones, directly on the most prominent bony points [referred to as the Anterior Superior Iliac Spine, or ASIS], and look straight down toward your feet. If one hand appears to be more forward than the other, that indicates pelvic rotation through the lumbar spine.)

Do you have high arches or flat feet? Are both feet the same?

Do either or both of your ankles roll inward/outward? (Hint: While keeping your toes and heels on the ground, try to rotate your ankle in each direction and notice the range of motion. For example, since my ankles are positioned inward, there is more range of motion outward.)

What direction do your knees point—straight ahead, inward, outward? Be aware that your left and right knees can point in different directions. (Hint: Look at the direction of your knee caps.)

Do your knees point in the same direction as your feet? (Note: As was discussed in the last chapter, knees and feet that point in different directions result in twisting at the knee.)

Do your knees line up with your ankles? Or are they inside your ankles, coming close together (knock kneed), or are they outside your ankles, moving away from each other (bow legged)?

Is your pelvis level right to left? (Hint: Look at the curve of your side from your pelvis to your armpit. If one side of your pelvis is higher, the curve will generally be more pronounced on that side.)

Is your rib cage centered in your torso, or is it shifted or rotated to one side?

body

Are your shoulders even? (Hint: Look at your hand position. If one hand is higher, that indicates an elevated shoulder.)

Is there equal space between your torso and your inner arm?

What part of your hand is facing forward—the back of the hand, the thumb, or somewhere in between? (Note: This is assessing rounding in your shoulders. The ideal position is with the thumb forward.)

Is your head balanced? (Hint: Look at your ears. If they are level, your head should be centered.)

Are your eyes in the same position and open evenly on each side?

Is there anything else that you notice about your front posture?

Side View Analysis

When looking at the body from the side, you are measuring your front-to-back balance. You are noticing the symmetry, or lack of symmetry, in the front and back halves of your body. Ideally, if you dropped a plumb line down your load-bearing joints—shoulders, hips, knees and ankles—the line would bisect each joint in the middle, and there would be an equal proportion of your body in front of and behind the line. It is not uncommon to have good side-to-side balance and poor front-to-back balance or vice-versa.

Step 1. Position Yourself

Stand sideways in front of a full-length mirror at ninety-degrees in a relaxed position, wearing minimal clothing and no shoes.

Step 2. Observe Your Posture

Record your answers in the space below each question or in your journal.

Are your ankles, knees and hips aligned? (Hint: Observe if your legs go straight down to the floor from your hips or if your lower legs go backward and hyperextend. If your heels come off the floor when you sit on the floor with your legs stretched out in front of you, thighs tightened, your lower leg is hyperextended.)

Do you have a big or small curve in your lower back? Mid-upper back? Neck? (Hint: *How do your curves compare with those that have ideal aligned posture in the last chapter [Figure 6-14]?* Check your lower back curve by lying in a 90-90 position on the ground, with your knees bent at ninety degrees and lower legs supported by a chair or couch. A lower back that does not touch the ground generally has an exaggerated lumbar curve.)

What is the tilt of your pelvis? Forward? Backward? (Note: A healthy pelvis tilts forward slightly. Recall the bowl of water analogy in the last chapter. A backward-tilting pelvis is less common in active people. If your pelvis is tilting back, you will likely notice a flatter lower back curve and a possible bend in your knees.)

Are your shoulders and hips positioned directly atop each other?

Is your head positioned forward, in front of your shoulders? (Hint: If you can't tell, stand with your back to the wall. Your heels, butt and upper back should touch the wall. Heels may be slightly away from the wall, depending on your structure. Move your feet away from the wall slightly if you feel like you are going to fall forward. Notice if your head also touches the wall naturally, without forcing a contraction in the upper body. If it does, your head and shoulders are aligned. If you have to raise your chin and tilt your head back to get your head on the wall, your head is forward.)

Is there anything else that you notice about your side posture?

body

Step 3. Draw it Out

Now that you've observed your posture in the mirror, keep a record of it by using the models in Figure 7-1. Your drawings don't have to be a work of art, but just enough to give you an idea of your current posture when you refer back to them. For simplicity, you could just mark the major deviations—the ones that stand out to you the most. Figure 7-2 provides examples of how to use the stick figure models. Alternatively, you could take your own posture pictures and draw lines through your ear (side view) and load-bearing joints—shoulders, hips, knees and ankles.

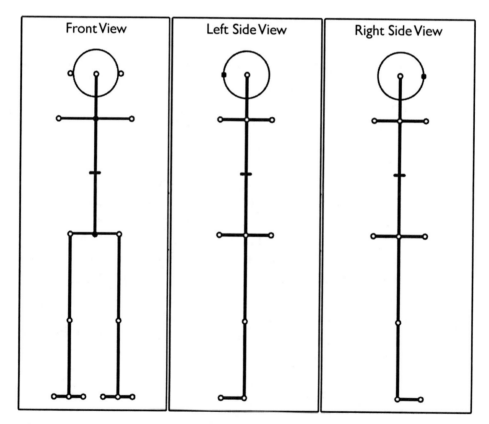

Figure 7-1. Mark the positions of your bones on the stick figure models—feet, knees, pelvis, spinal curves, rib cage, shoulders and head—to create a representation of your posture.

Front View

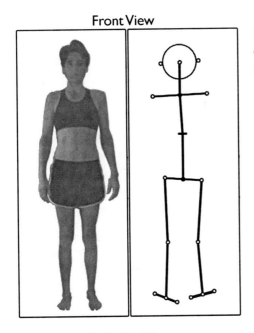

Figure 7-2. Examples of how to complete the stick figure models using my posture photos.

body

Left Side View   Right Side View

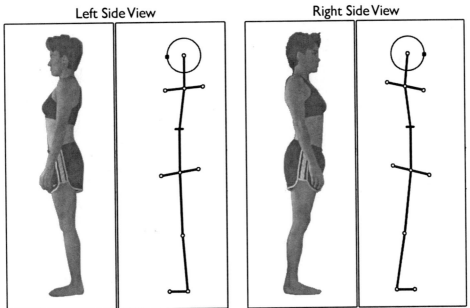

Step 4. Balance Test

To conclude your static posture self-assessment, let's do a balance test. Your feet are the contact points with the ground and tell you a lot about what is going on with your alignment above. Evenly contacting feet reflect a symmetrical skeleton. With your shoes off, stand on a hard surface in your natural, relaxed posture with your eyes closed. Feel how your weight is distributed throughout your feet—left to right, front to back and side to side. Make note of your weight distribution on Figure 7-3. An example is provided in Figure 7-4.

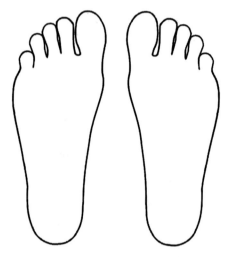 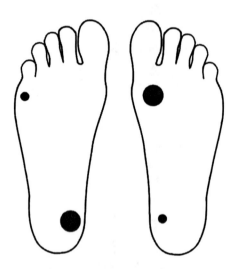

Figure 7-3. Mark where you feel the heaviest contact in your feet with the ground.

Figure 7-4. Example of the weight distribution through my feet, the larger dots indicating heavier contact.

Motion Self-Assessments

Now we're going to examine some additional factors that will provide information about what happens when you're moving. These self-assessments will give you an idea of how the forces are being directed through your body, starting at the feet.

Foot and Shoe Wear

Let's take a close look at your feet and notice how they are being used in and out of your shoes. Here are a few more questions for you.

Do you have bunions? Are they the same on the left and right?

Do your toes all point straight ahead? Or do some overlap? Or do some bend in or out?

Are there areas of continuous redness on your feet?

Do you have hard calluses on your feet? Corns? Blisters? Are they symmetrical side to side?

Have you suffered a Morton's neuroma or other foot problems?

Is there anything else that you notice about your feet?

body

I know a lot of people will say many of these conditions are hereditary: "My mom (or sister, dad, uncle, etc.) had this, so I do, too." These conditions *may* be passed down through the generations, but they are not necessarily genetic. Rather, they may be the result of modeling the behaviors and movements of adults in a child's environment. According to Albert Bandura, Ph.D., a social cognitive psychologist and Professor Emeritus at Stanford, children learn by imitating others. This concept of "observational learning" is fundamental to Bandura's "social learning theory."[2] Early in life, when we're acquiring movement skills, we copy the biomechanics of the adults around us—the good ones and the bad ones. I don't want to discount these familial influences on the development of some conditions, but I also believe there is a postural component that can be addressed.

Here's an example: I have a large bunion on my right foot, and I have learned that it is a consequence of my faulty gait mechanics. While walking, instead of extending my foot and toes to push off, I twist my ankle out sideways, putting a lot of pressure on the bunion area of my foot when I take a step. My dad also has bunions and

139

other foot issues. So, I may have learned my poor stride from him. However, I have noticed that my bunion and the associated pain have reduced as my posture and gait mechanics have improved. Perhaps my dad's bunions would have also reduced with a more balanced structure and walk.

Now let's look at your shoes. The sole of your shoe can indicate a great deal about how you're striking the ground when engaged in a repetitive-motion, weight-bearing sport, such as running, walking or hiking. Grab a pair of your well-worn favorites, and record your findings under each question, in your journal, or at the end of the chapter.

Hold up both shoes with the sole side up. Look at the wear patterns on the left shoe versus the right. *What do you notice? Is there more wear at the front/back/inside/outside? How do the left and right shoes compare?*

Next, turn both shoes over and notice the integrity of the shoe around the toe box, the heel, and both sides. *What do you notice? Is one area of the shoe breaking down more than the other? Is one shoe—left versus right—wearing differently than the other?*

Now take each shoe individually and look at the wear on the inside of the shoe—around the heel cup, throughout the top and bottom of the shoe, and on both sides. This is especially important for non-weight-bearing repetitive sports like cycling, where the sole of the shoe isn't going to provide much information. *Is there any asymmetrical wear on the insides of your shoes?*

Any differences in your feet or shoes—left to right, front to back, side to side, or top to bottom—are indicators of uneven use. Blisters, bunions, hammer toes, plantar fasciitis, and many other issues can all be signs of movement discrepancies.[3] This was the case for my husband, Ken.

Ken often develops blisters on his right heel during long hikes. Previous right knee surgeries have altered his walking pattern on this side of his body. His right foot points out when he strides, whereas his left points straight. The unbalanced movements in his hip, knee, and upper leg travel down his lower leg, affecting his foot strike and gait. This creates friction and a resultant blister on the back of his heel. Examination of his shoes, both sport and dress, show increased signs of wear on the inner right heel.

NOTE: As far as musculoskeletal function is concerned, having the same problem on both feet or shoes is actually a good sign because it is probably just the result of poor footwear.

Unilateral Muscle Soreness

It is common to be sore after activity, especially if you haven't done it recently or are pushing your distance or intensity. The soreness you feel, however, should be symmetrical. If one hamstring, hip, or shoulder is consistently tighter than the other after playing your sport, this tightness is a concern. It is likely that you are moving differently on your right and left sides during the activity. The human body is a bilateral machine, so each side should be used equally. *Do you have unilateral muscle soreness?*

Repeat Injuries on the Same Side

Clients often tell me that all of their pain and repetitive injuries occur on one side of their body, from their head to their toes. Having had three left knee surgeries and one left hip surgery, I can relate. It is obviously not that the left side of my body is older than the right, even though my clients often blame their pain on advancing age. Rather, the left and right sides were not moving in harmony. Because of the compromised position and biomechanics of my left side, it was overstressed, and it broke down. *Are your injuries all on the same side?*

Uneven Muscle Development

My left calf is bigger than my right. This is a sign of unbalanced movements. When I'm out on the trails, in the gym or on the slopes, I'm not using my body symmetrically. My left calf, it turns out, has taken over

body

doing the work for my left gluteal muscles. More on this in Chapter 8. *Do you notice uneven muscle development?*

Postural Awareness Aids Healing

Now that you have greater understanding of the position and function of your body, you can use this information to your advantage to accelerate your recovery. As they say, *knowledge is power!* Connecting with your body and gaining greater awareness of your structure is the first step toward healing.

To help raise a client's body awareness of her current alignment, I begin with a posture assessment, similar to what you just did. I often take photos of the client's static posture from the front, back and both sides. These images are often enlightening. Many clients have no idea what their bodies really look like. When they see the structural analysis, many for the first time, clients start to understand how their posture and pain are related and what needs to change for healing. This awareness alone is empowering. By knowing what needs to change, you can make adjustments throughout your day that can bring relief. Greater consciousness of your body can also impact your mental and emotional states, as my client Bernice explains:

Jessica's first step was helping me recognize my problems. She started with my posture. I thought it was pretty good, that I had better than average body awareness, and that I stood up straight. On closer inspection I learned that my right shoulder was in front of the left, my weight was off centered toward my right leg, my right foot turned out, and my hips and shoulders weren't level.

After I became somewhat aware of my body misalignments, the next step was to determine what I could do to correct this. Jessica guided me to these "ah ha" moments where I could feel the imbalance. Then she taught me how to relax the overused muscles and strengthen underused muscles. In time my right foot turned forward, my body weight moved toward the center of my body, and my hip pain disappeared.

Since then, Jessica has helped me also "see" my shoulders in a new way. As a computer scientist, I had abused my upper body by sitting in a chair, typing away, hour after hour. The pain would radiate through my shoulder, into my back, down into my fingertips, and up into my neck. One tactic Jessica used while working with me was to have me use my rhomboids [muscles between the shoulder blades and spine] to pull my shoulders back. I didn't realize how to move these muscles, so she coached me by placing her hand on my back and noting when they tightened. It felt great. I was putting muscles in motion that hadn't moved in a long time.

I began to expand my specific muscle awareness repertoire. I'm less likely to catch myself in a "C" shape posture, Figure 7-5(b). For example, I remember one time sitting in a crowded room on top of a table that, of course, had no back support. I was slouched and my back was hurting. When I realized what I was doing and that I was strong enough to sit up straight, Figure 7-5(a), I found I was more comfortable doing so. I knew that I had a lasting change in my posture.

Increasing my body awareness has dramatically impacted my quality of life. Sure, I still hurt sometimes, but I eventually understood what causes it, how to prevent it, and how to correct it. Also, I'm less likely to injure myself because I'm paying more attention, I'm more agile, and my body dynamics are better balanced. Because I catch my destructive actions sooner, treat them quicker and recover faster, I have less pain. I've gone from being unaware of issues to correcting them, from pain to relief, from muscle tension to comfortable stability, from injury to agility, from desperate to hopeful, and from fear to confidence and better judgment.

Learning to pay attention to this body has helped me emotionally, mentally and physically. The closer I pay attention, the more at peace I am. I

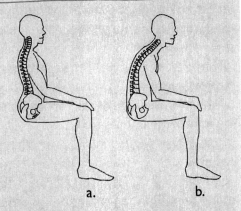

Figure 7-5. (a) Healthy spine alignment has three curves, alternating from the low back, up to the mid-back, and then to the neck. (b) Rounded spine alignment resembles the letter "C." In the "C" posture, all of the curves are going in the same direction, rounding forward.

body

live here, and when I'm aware, I learn about my body AND mind and soul. This pile of flesh guides me through my life in a much healthier, peaceful mode if I listen. Beyond mental and emotional guidance, I've learned, too, that if I look at my pain, I can learn from it. Not just how to alleviate it but also to see the error of my ways. In reality, my body is a guide to a closer walk with my heart.

How Did Your Body Get Askew?

If you're like most active people, your self-assessment revealed unbalanced posture. Your joints were not all perfectly lined up, and the weight in your feet was not even. It's impossible to know how long your body has been in this position. Muscle imbalances that generate postural asymmetries, as you will learn in Chapter 8, have several sources, including a sedentary lifestyle, repetitive sports, habitual daily living movement patterns, and previous injuries.[1]

You are a collection of your experiences, injuries, and habits. What you do throughout your day greatly impacts your muscular balance. Take a look at the positions you're in during the day, and you might begin to see how those habits are impacting your skeletal position. Are you standing on one foot more often? Do you spend hours hunched over a computer? Do you always cross your right leg over your left when sitting or vice versa? What is your sleeping position? How do you carry things—purses, backpacks, children? These are all factors to consider in determining how your muscles have become imbalanced.

It's also likely you had at least one injury—maybe more—earlier in your life that contributed to your current alignment. When you're hurt, you start moving differently to protect the injured part and to limit pain. Just think about how you might hop around if you sprained your ankle, broke your leg or had knee pain. Even as the pain is diminishing and you begin using your legs more evenly, there may be subtle imbalances in your motion. Unfortunately, these uneven movement patterns are often unknowingly maintained, even once the pain has gone. Add onto this another injury and more movement modifications, and your motion and your function further decline. With each episode of pain and injury, another layer of movement accommodation and postural imbalance is added.

Pain and trauma also contribute to muscle imbalances by affecting a muscle's ability to engage. Dr. Marc Heller, DC, who specializes in back pain, explains: "Any pain that lasts more than 48 hours begins to alter function. That means trigger points begin to develop, the pain spreads up and down the chain, and key stability muscles shut down."[4] When key stability muscles shut down, you are primed for overuse and compensation by the surrounding joints and muscles, which may need to take on greater stability roles, sacrificing mobility in the process. Recall from Chapter 5 that each joint is designed to be both mobile and stable. You don't want to give up either.

Despite your development of postural asymmetries, your body continues to respond to the demands you place on it. It does this for a long time, growing more and more imbalanced in the process. There comes a point, right now perhaps, when your body cannot continue to compensate its way around functional movement and forces you to stop. This downward progression needs to be reversed. It is the subject of the next chapter.

Injury-Proof Your Body

When working with clients, I'm generally not so interested in the details of how their injuries occurred, such as unraveling how their bodies became cockeyed. Rather, I just want to help them move forward in their healing. Often, the injury was caused by a combination of factors that can be difficult to separate out. Instead of dwelling on the past, I encourage my clients to look toward the future. For many clients, though, the specifics of how the injury happened are important to them, and they need to talk it out, so I listen closely. The injury story I hear focuses on the external movement pattern that caused pain: twisting when lifting, jumping down, squatting, running uphill, reaching up into a cabinet, swimming butterfly, and so on. In the client's view, it was something they did, a specific motion that generated the agony. However, I respectfully disagree. The movement was what *triggered* the pain, what broke the camel's back, if you will, but there were underlying causes—such as muscle imbalances, posture misalignments, strength disparities, inefficient movement mechanics, lack of mobility or stability—that predisposed the client to injury. The offending movement was just what pushed the body over the edge and caused the pain. In my opinion, the injury resulted not from the activity itself, but how the activity was performed. Recall that it is the *position and condition* of the body brought into movement that matters the most. As an alignment coach, I want to know, did the body cheat to move? Is the body lacking appropriate function to execute the maneuver correctly?

If you feel it was the activity that created your pain, I have some questions for you. Had you done that activity before without pain? Do other people do that movement without pain? If so, is it really the movement that is the problem? Probably not. Unfortunately, many of us do blame the activity for our injury, so we develop a strategy of avoidance. There is now a fear of pain associated with the activity, so we protect ourselves from further discomfort by avoiding the offending movement. Many clients tell me, "I don't run because it hurts my [back, hip, knee . . . fill in the blank]." Yes, running—or any activity, for that matter—hurts when done in a compromised position and when using poor form, but this can be changed. If you eliminate an activity every time there is pain, you will eventually have a very small circle of non-threatening movements and sports. But pain now during an activity does not mean pain forever. *You can be active without pain!* Broaden your sports circle; don't let it close in around you. Make your body injury-proof for the future. The first step toward this goal is improving your body alignment and function. The next chapter shows you how.

Summary

Misaligned posture may be the root of your chronic pain. Static posture tells a story about how you are using your body when you move and play sports. If you are out of alignment standing still, these muscle imbalances will carry over into your activities, causing lopsided movement patterns that can lead to injury and pain. Asymmetrical wear on your feet and shoes, unilateral muscle soreness, repeat injuries on the same side of your body, and uneven muscle development are all signs that you are not moving symmetrically.

Awareness of your posture is empowering, not only in body but also in mind. Having a greater understanding of your position allows you to take immediate action in healing your pain and preventing another injury. There could be many reasons you developed muscle imbalances and crooked posture, but those reasons should not be your main concern. Focus your efforts on moving forward from where you are and gaining better alignment now to prolong and expand your athletics for your future.

body

Game Winning Strategies

Additional copies of the self-assessment tools—stick figure models, foot outlines, motion self-assessment charts—are available for download on my website: www.thepfathlete.com/resources.

1. ### Complete the Posture Self-Assessment

    If you haven't done the self-assessment, schedule some time to go through the analysis before moving on to the next chapter.

2. ### Complete the Motion Self-Assessments

    Record your findings below or in your journal.

Foot and shoe wear
Unilateral muscle soreness
Repeat injuries on the same side
Uneven muscle development

body

8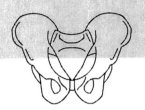

Balancing Postural Deviations

So, how did your posture self-assessment turn out? Are you straight as an arrow with no need to read further? Or did you find some postural issues? If you're like me, prior to critically looking at your posture, it probably never occurred to you that the position of your bones was a problem. You may not have considered that structural changes in your alignment could be contributing to your chronic pain or raising your risk of injury. I was stubborn, and despite the clear evidence of my postural asymmetries, I still didn't understand how this related to my chronic pain. Even after paying a large sum of money for 16 Egoscue Method® posture therapy sessions, I remained skeptical. It took a major shift in my thinking to overcome my resistance and commit to Egoscue Method® posture therapy, a seemingly subtle and yet radically different approach to healing. However, although I was out of my comfort zone with this approach, lacking other options, I persisted with the therapy. The turning point for me, what convinced me that Egoscue Method® posture therapy was what I should do, came when I intellectually grasped the theory behind the exercises. I needed to know the *"why?"* Just as I talked about knowing *why* you hurt in Chapter 5, I needed to know the *why* behind my posture asymmetries and how these simple exercises were going to correct the problem. I was still clinging to my "no pain, no gain," "more is better," and "it has to hurt and be hard to be effective" mindset.

That's what this chapter is about, giving you the *why* behind the postural deviations you saw in the last chapter. Generally, the downward postural cascade to asymmetry starts with muscle imbalances, which progress to become dysfunctions that lead to compensations.[1]

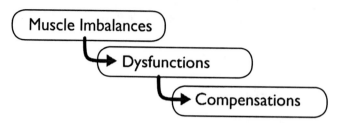

I'll start the discussion at the beginning with muscle imbalances.

Muscle Imbalances

The position of your skeleton is maintained through soft tissues—muscles, tendons, ligaments and connective tissues, including the myofascia. All of these soft tissues are involved in joint position. For simplicity, I am going to use the familiar terms—muscle imbalances and balanced muscles—to refer to all of these structures for this discussion. Balanced muscles maintain correct joint alignment. Postural asymmetries, then, indicate the presence of muscle imbalances.[1]

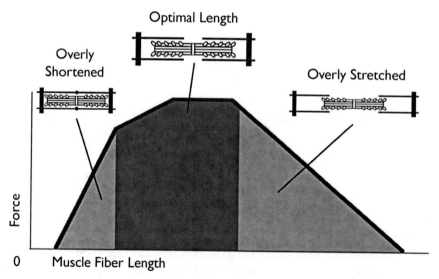

Figure 8-1. There is a length-tension relationship between the position of a muscle and the force it can produce.[2] Muscle loses strength when it is too long or too short.

152

In addition to muscle imbalances, postural asymmetries also indicate weakness. The strength of a muscle depends on its resting length and tension. Muscle force is generated when the protein fibers—actin (thin outer fibers) and myosin (thick inner fiber)—within the muscle cells slide past and bind to one another, known as the "sliding filament theory."[2] In order to generate optimal force, muscle cells need to be at a normal, or slightly longer than normal, resting length without excessive tension. Too much overlap between the muscle protein fibers when the muscle is shortened, or too little overlap when the muscle is lengthened, results in reduced force production, or failure of the muscle to perform the requested movement, as shown in Figure 8-1.[2]

If postural deviations indicate muscle imbalances and display weakness, *I was weak!* As an example, let's consider my rounded posture through my mid-upper back and shoulders, as shown in Figure 8-2.

In this overly-flexed upper body position, there is shortening and tightening of the muscles in the front of the shoulder, around the chest, and into the anterior neck. There is also lengthening and tightening of the muscles in the upper back and posterior neck. Short and long muscles can be tight, and both are weak. Read that again: *short and long muscles can be tight, and both are weak.*

Just by looking at my upper body postural deviations, you can surmise that I had weakness in the muscles on both sides of my shoulders. From my static posture, you could also correctly infer that I had excessive tension in these muscles. These weaknesses and tensions contributed to my chronic pain. Analyzing static alignment exposes postural asymmetries that have resulted from muscle imbalances. Standing postural assessment is a powerful tool that can reveal information about how your body is functioning and why you might hurt, as you discovered in Chapter 7.

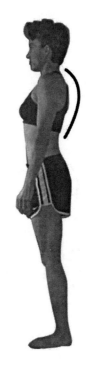

body

Figure 8-2. Muscle imbalances between the front and back of the body create postural asymmetries in the side view.

Beware of Stretching Your Hamstrings

Muscles need to be balanced between the front and back as well as the left and right sides of the body to maintain aligned posture. Aside from the rounding of the upper body, another common postural imbalance is typically seen at the pelvis. The hip flexors (at the front of the body) and the hamstrings (at the back of the body) work in opposition to hold the pelvis in a neutral position, as shown in Figure 8-3(a). In my posture (Figure 8-2), and in many of my athletic clients, the hip flexors are tight and short, pulling the pelvis too far forward, which creates extra length and tension in the hamstrings, as shown in Figure 8-3(b).

In this scenario the hamstrings are too long and tight. The last thing they need is to be stretched and lengthened farther. But of course, that's exactly what many of us do, including me. Feeling tightness in the muscles on the back of my thighs and being ingrained with the notion that hamstrings

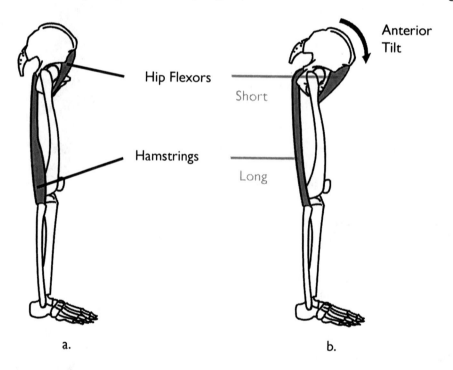

a.   b.

Figure 8-3. (a) A neutral pelvis position with balanced hip flexors and hamstrings. (b) A forward-tilted pelvis with tight, short and weak hip flexors opposing tight, long and weak hamstrings.

always need to be stretched, I regularly over-lengthened these muscles with deep stretches. If you stretch an already lengthened rubber band, what happens? Greater tension develops, and it is more likely to break. Hamstring strain, anyone?

Functional hamstring length is 90-degrees,[3] as I will demonstrate in the next section. When you go much beyond this, it can lead to problems with stability, proprioception and muscle usage. Having overstretched hamstrings was one of my major alignment issues, which I will discuss in Chapter 11.

Test Your Hamstring Length

This test is best done with a partner, but it can also be done alone. Lie on your back with your legs straight. Without bending your knee, lift your leg up, bringing it as close to your torso as possible. If you have a partner, he will place one hand on the back of your ankle and the other just above your knee in the front, as shown in Figure 8-4. Stretch the leg as far as you can while keeping the knee locked straight. Stop when you feel increased tension and resistance to further movement. If you can raise your leg up to 90-degrees, perpendicular to the

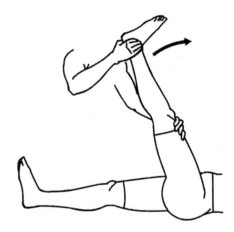

Figure 8-4. Healthy hamstring length is 90-degrees with your knee straight.

ground, you have ample hamstring length. I cringe when I see people in my posture classes or during private sessions who can pull their legs up toward their ears or bend over and palm the floor with their hands. I just know from experience where that over-flexibility can lead. If your hamstrings went past 100-degrees, they are considered to be dysfunctional muscles, which will be discussed shortly in relation to the hip flexors and glutes. I will also talk specifically about dysfunctional hamstrings in Chapter 11.

body

Reposition Your Pelvis to Release Your Hamstrings

The position of your pelvis, to which your hamstrings connect, influences the outcome of your hamstring length test. If the results of your hamstring length test showed short or long hamstrings, consider following the recommended strategy below to reposition your pelvis. After implementation of the strategy, repeat the test to check for improvement and verification of the intervention. You may find that a combination of both strategies is most effective, especially if your hamstrings are too long.

Strategy 1: Short Hamstrings

First, let me clarify that if you found that one or both of your hamstrings did not reach 90-degrees, it doesn't necessarily mean that your hamstrings are short if your pelvis is in a forwardly tilted position. Overly tight hip flexors can hold the pelvis forward. Although the hamstring muscles may be at a proper length and tension, they will *appear* short in the hamstring length test due to the anterior tilt of the pelvis. In many athletes the hip flexors, which are heavily used in sports, are short and tight. In this case, the length of the hip flexors needs to be increased. Figure 8-5 shows a common stretch for the hip flexors.

Kneeling Hip Flexor Stretch

You can watch a video of this exercise on my website: www.thepfathlete.com/resources.

1. Start in a kneeling position, with your forward leg bent at 90-degree angles from your hip to your knee and from your knee to your ankle, Figure 8-5(a). Be sure your front foot is positioned straight and that the weight is equally distributed throughout your foot. Position your back foot so that it is turned under and relaxed. This is best felt with bare feet.

2. Your back leg is also at a 90-degree angle, with your thigh perpendicular to the ground.

3. Ensure that your upper body is aligned directly above your back leg, with a straight line from your shoulder to your knee.

4. Place your hands on your forward leg without twisting your upper body.

5. Maintain this alignment while you tuck your pelvis under to lengthen the front of your hip. This is where you should feel the stretch.

6. To increase the intensity of the stretch, lean your whole body forward, keeping the alignment from your shoulder to knee, Figure 8-5(b).

7. Once you have moved forward, re-tuck your pelvis under.

8. Breathe in through your nose and out through your mouth as you hold this position for one to two minutes.

body

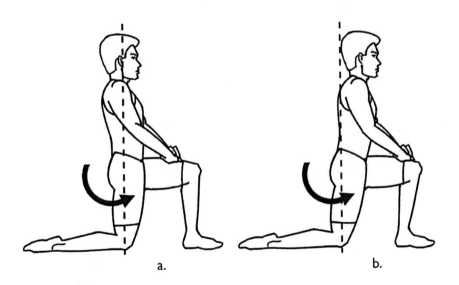

a. b.

Figure 8-5. The kneeling hip flexor stretch releases tension in the hip flexors to allow the pelvis to rotate backward (posterior tilt, indicated by the arrows) into a more neutral posture, which repositions the hamstrings.

Strategy 2: Long Hamstrings

If you found that one or both of your hamstrings easily surpassed 90-degrees, you probably need to strengthen, and thus shorten, your hamstrings.[4] Here's another thing to consider: If your leg went way beyond 90-degrees and your pelvis was tilted forward when you did the hamstring test, this means that your hamstrings are actually even longer than they would be if your pelvis were neutral. *Thus, you really need to shorten your hamstrings!* So, although it may seem counter intuitive to strengthen the hamstrings when they feel tight, this is often precisely what is needed. The hamstring muscle in Figure 8-3(b) feels tight because it is too long. The pelvis has tipped forward and has pulled the hamstring with it. By strengthening your hamstrings with a shortening contraction, you can pull the pelvis back and release tension on the hamstring muscles, as shown in the bridge exercise (Figure 8-6). The hamstrings are important players in core alignment and breathing, as you'll learn in Chapter 10.

Hamstring and Glute Bridge

You can watch a video of this exercise on my website:
www.thepfathlete.com/resources.

1. Lie on the ground with your knees bent at 90 degrees and your upper body relaxed, arms out to your sides with your palms up, Figure 8-6(a).

2. Maintain sensory awareness of your heels and big toes without pushing into the ground for proper alignment of the feet, knees and hips. There is a tendency for the feet to roll out, which is why you need to keep the big toes down. This is best felt with bare feet.

3. Inhale. Then, as you exhale, flatten your back by gently tilting your pelvis up toward your head. Push your knees forward slightly to engage your deep transverse abdominis (TA) muscle. Avoid over-contracting your rectus abdominis ("six-pack muscle"). Keep this muscle relaxed, Figure 8-6(b). This is the initial movement of

the pelvic tilt exercise described in Chapter 9. Maintain this position throughout the exercise.

4. Pull back into your heels to engage your hamstrings, and lift your hips off the ground by using your glutes, Figure 8-6(c). In this position you should feel your hamstrings and glutes working. Without allowing your lower back to overly arch, keep the activation in your abdominals to ensure that you maintain good alignment through your torso.

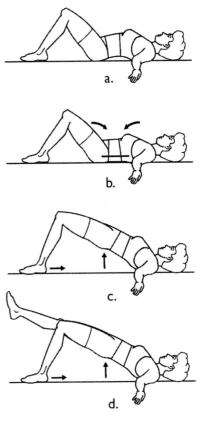

5. Breathe in through your nose and out through your mouth as you hold the position for a minute.

   NOTE: If only one hamstring was overly flexible, you will want to lift the opposite foot off the ground to bias the exercise to that side, Figure 8-6(d). For example, if your left hamstring went farther beyond 90-degrees, you will want to lift your right foot off the ground to make the left side work harder. Watch that your pelvis stays steady and doesn't move as you do this. You will need to push more into the ground with your supporting leg in order to hold your alignment. If lifting the leg is too challenging, start by raising your heel and going up on your toe.

   Figure 8-6. The hamstring and glute bridge shortens the length of the hamstrings by rotating the pelvis backward into a neutral posture.

6. Repeat one or two more times.

body

Dysfunctions

Muscle and joint dysfunctions tend to occur when there are muscle imbalances. Dysfunction simply means that the muscle or joint is not performing the work for which it is designed.[1] For example, my overstretched upper back and shoulder muscles were no longer doing their job to extend my upper back and hold my shoulder blades in a balanced position. Rather, they were stuck in a tight and long orientation, creating a rounded posture. These muscles had become dysfunctional. In this situation, the shoulder joint can also become dysfunctional because it cannot move in a full range of motion as a result of its compromised position.

When muscles are held in a shortened or lengthened position for an extended period, this modified posture can become the new normal. The nervous system, which directs muscle action and coordinates movement, adapts to maintain this new, although compromised, posture, by influencing muscle tone (tension). As I learned through my studies at Egoscue University®, "Muscles become dysfunctional when length-tension relationships become altered (e.g. shortened, lengthened, tight, loose). This has an impact on the proper rate of contraction and sequencing, resulting in inefficient and/or uncoordinated movement."[1] Consequently, alignment and movement are altered with muscle dysfunctions.

A common muscle dysfunction occurs across the hip joint, between the gluteal muscles and hip flexors, which work in opposition to each other, as shown in Figure 8-7.

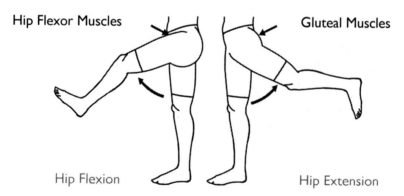

Figure 8-7. Hip flexors bend the hip, bringing the thigh closer to the front of the torso, while the gluteal muscles extend the hip, bringing the thigh farther from the front of the torso.

Not only did I have this dysfunction, but I have also seen it in many of my clients. Tight hip flexors, in addition to tilting the pelvis too far forward and possibly over-lengthening the hamstrings as was just discussed, can also impair gluteal function. Since the hip flexors on the front of the body are short and tight, the gluteal muscles on the back of the body tend to be long and tight, just like the hamstrings. Because of their imbalanced positions, neither group of muscles—hip flexors nor glutes—are generally strong or working optimally. However, in my case, my glutes, particularly those on my left side where I had more pain and trauma, were barely working at all. My inability to contract my left glutes was partially due to my exceptionally tight left hip flexors on the front side of my body. I know this sounds really technical. The only reason I'm going into all of this detail is because I see it so often in my clients, and it might be happening to you. I'll continue to explain.

Together, the brain and spinal cord form the central nervous system (CNS), which directs the muscles to move the bones. So, the brain sends messages down the spinal cord through the nerves (motor neurons); these nerves tell muscles what to do; and muscles tell bones what to do (Figure 8-8).[5]

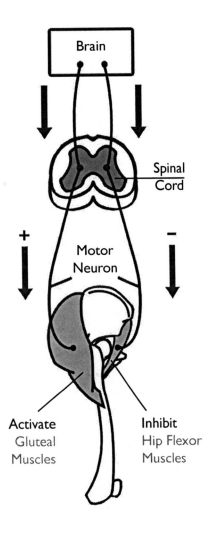

Figure 8-8. Muscles on opposing sides of the hip joint are activated or inhibited through nerve impulses that originate in the brain.

body

Since hip flexion and extension cannot be performed simultaneously, one muscle is stimulated to move, while the other is inhibited from contracting, as shown in Figure 8-8. This is known as reciprocal inhibition.[6] When a muscle group has too much tension, in this case the hip flexors, it becomes more sensitive to nerve stimulation and basically takes all of the nerve impulse for itself so that the opposing muscle group, in this case the gluteal muscles, doesn't receive a signal to engage.[6]

When I attempted to activate my gluteal muscles correctly during a hip extension exercise, my overly tight hip flexors would fire prematurely, and my glutes didn't tighten. *My butt muscles never got the message to engage!* With repetition, this pattern became stronger, and my glutes became weaker. I have found dysfunctional glutes to be the source of many ailments related to pelvic position with my clients, including sciatica, back pain, sacroiliac joint (SIJ) dysfunction, hip bursitis, tailbone pain and much more. Dysfunctional glutes can even be contributing to your neck pain and bunions. (Recall that I had both of these.) Your glutes are critically important to your pelvic position. Also, as you'll learn in Chapter 9, your pelvis is a foundational piece of your core. If this central structure is not aligned and solid, dysfunction and pain can spread throughout the body.

Compensations

Compensations follow muscle imbalances and dysfunctions. Your body is always trying to help you and to facilitate your ability to do what you want, regardless of your dysfunction. If you want to swim, your body will do its best to figure out a movement sequence and then will fire muscles to make that happen. It may not be pretty or mechanically efficient, but your body will get the job done. In doing so, however, your body will likely compensate. When one body part—muscle or joint—is recruited to do the work for a dysfunctional body part, this is known as a compensation.[1]

If you refer back to my previous example, I was dysfunctional in my hamstrings and glutes and couldn't use them to extend my hip. Therefore, my body had to compensate and figure out another way to move my leg backward. And it did—by using my lower back muscles and extending (arching) my lumbar spine. That might be why your back hurts during activities that require hip extension. I commonly see this with clients who classic cross-country ski and run. Because the back is compensating for the glutes, chronic pain develops with the activity. Hamstrings can also compensate by taking on a greater role in hip extension when the glutes are weak. This is a double whammy on the hamstrings, which are often positioned too long and tight and are now being overused for hip extension. *Ouch!*

Up to this point in my discussion about dysfunctions and compensations, I have kept the conversation mostly focused on muscles. However, dysfunctions and compensations also affect the joints. Using my client Tarik from Chapter 5 as my example, his tight hips were dysfunctional. They couldn't move properly, so his adjacent joints—knees and low back—compensated. These stability dominant joints—knees and low back—increased their mobility to the point of becoming damaged and painful themselves. Additionally, tight and misaligned hip joints cannot accept load well—even gravity and body weight—and rely on the surrounding joints to absorb more of the force.

This is what our bodies do to allow us to perform, despite our dysfunctions: they compensate, often without our realizing it. However, the body can only compensate for so long before it starts to breakdown and hurt. Over time, and with repetition, these poor biomechanics take a toll on our bodies, and we feel pain. At this point, it is up to us to listen to these signals and act accordingly to respect our bodies and minimize injury.

body

Re-aligning the Body

If ending my pain was just a matter of correcting my muscle imbalances and moving the bones back into place, *why didn't I have better success with stretching my hip flexors, getting massage and seeing a chiropractor?* As I've explained, stretching my hip flexors should lengthen the front of my hip and allow my pelvis to tilt backward into a more neutral posture. Massage was treating my soft tissue discrepancies—releasing built up tension, allowing bones to reposition, and improving circulation. Also, the chiropractor was adjusting my skeleton. Through manipulation, she was moving my bones and putting my joints back into ideal alignment. Additionally, she explained to me how this was also resetting my nervous system to enable appropriate muscle firing patterns. Together this seemed the ideal combination for healing. But long term, it wasn't working.

My clients have similar experiences, telling me how much better they feel after these restorative treatments, how their symptoms just disappear. Their bliss is only temporary, though. Shortly after they go back to their normal activities, the pain returns. *Why?* Manipulating the bones and soft tissues into the correct position feels good, but it is not re-educating the soft tissue function to allow the body to maintain the new alignment. Consequently, the results are fleeting. Once we start moving again in our typical, uneven and compensated patterns, the soft tissues revert back to asymmetrical positions, our posture returns to its lopsided state, and our pain comes back.

Your body needs stability. Stability is gained when structures of your body contact or impinge on one another. For instance, stability comes from the ground up, happening when the ankle bones stack appropriately on top of each other to support your structure.[7] If you tend to walk on the outside edge of your foot, your foot bones don't touch on the inside, which creates instability in your foot and throughout your body. A good way to test this is to notice if you can feel your heel through your big toe when you walk, which is necessary for proper gait mechanics. (Read more about this in Chapter 11.)

If your body cannot attain stability through correct impingement—for example, if those ankle bones are not properly stacked—it will improvise, often through incorrect impingement and contraction of muscles to hold areas of the body rigid.[7] Neck and shoulder tightness is a common way to stabilize the jaw and head position. So, in a strange way, your body *wants* the tightness that you just had released through chiropractic, massage, and stretching. And, if your body is not shown another way to gain stability, it will revert back to the old, painful pattern. This is also why your muscles remain tight, even though you may stretch every day. In your current alignment, they need to be tight to give you stability. They won't let go until another source of support is created.[7]

Repeatedly stretching my hip flexors, receiving massages and manipulating my joints into alignment kept me active for a time, but it wasn't fixing the underlying problem. Also, I wasn't doing anything to re-train my body to stay in the corrected position or to regain proper movement mechanics. I was still only addressing symptoms with these modalities. I hadn't gone deep enough to consider *why* my body stayed tight and misaligned. I hadn't discovered the mechanism that was causing the ongoing torque and tension throughout my structure. There are always reasons for muscle tightness and postural deviations. Both are signs of poor functional mechanics, which will only be exaggerated with the increased demands of sport. It is not normal or healthy to have consistent, excessive tightness in your body.

Passively putting the body parts back into place through the modalities described—massage, chiropractic and stretching—does not ensure they will stay there and start functioning properly. Most likely, the body has been moving incorrectly for a long time. There are layers of dysfunction and compensation patterns that need to be broken down before proper motion can be re-established. Some muscles need to be strengthened, while others need to relax. Long-lasting chronic pain relief can only be achieved through a program that both repositions and re-educates the soft tissues throughout the body. Since muscles move the bones, this can be accomplished through corrective postural exercises, such as the hamstring and glute bridge (Figure 8-6). This exercise is repositioning the pelvis while simultaneously re-educating the hamstrings and gluteal muscles so the body can maintain this new, aligned posture.

I'm not suggesting you stop chiropractic, stretching or massage; I personally use and endorse all of these modalities. Rather, I am advocating for the addition of muscle re-training to your routine so that your chiropractic adjustments hold longer, your massages are more beneficial, and you are confident that the stretches you are doing are appropriate for your body. Complementing these modalities with corrective posture exercises has been effective for me and my clients.

As my massage therapist Susan had suggested, faulty posture was holding me back from recovering. Posture was the larger issue that I couldn't identify when talking to my orthopedic surgeon about my recurring knee injuries. The overall position and lack of function throughout my body was playing an integral role in my ongoing pain. Although I was doing everything I thought I should to heal, there was a missing piece in my approach.

body

The Missing Piece: Muscle Re-training

Muscle re-training means going back to the basics of movement. The body is fantastic at enabling us to continue to play, regardless of our dysfunctions, by using compensations. And the fitter you are, the stronger and more ingrained these compensation patterns become. *Sorry!* This just means you will have to unlearn some old habits before embarking on developing new ones. It's not that hard, but it does take time, dedication, and patience. However, *you can do it!*

To strip down motion to its basics, you'll need to isolate movements. I know what you might be thinking: I've talked all about how the body works as a unit, and now I want to break up the kinetic chain. However, when re-learning motion, you need to take it apart so that when you put it back together, each link in the chain is working as designed. You want to ensure correct and functional mechanics, not a dysfunctional and compensated flow of movement.

When I teach a new student a simple knee pillow squeeze exercise, she often finds it difficult to isolate the muscle engagement to the inner thighs. Instead, her body will bring in the abdominals, neck, shoulders, or any other muscles that are willing to help into the movement. Often the body has become very good at engaging everything at the same time, making it hard to isolate one area. Consequently, that is *exactly* what you need to do to regain strength and function in that part of the body. If you consistently engage multiple muscles together, the weaker ones in the kinetic chain may fail to grow stronger as the other muscles compensate for their dysfunction. I'll be honest: corrective posture exercises aren't nearly as fun as playing sports. However, if you cannot do the basic movements and fundamental exercises correctly—using the right muscles for the right movement in the right order—you can bet you'll cheat with compensations when performing more complex, whole body activities. As I learned with running, your muscular and joint dysfunctions and movement compensations often propagate into your sports technique.

Through my recovery, the ongoing tightness in my lower back created pain when I was in the cycling position. To keep active, I tried running and found that it was a more acceptable movement to my body—or so I thought. I didn't have any lower body discomfort when I ran. Hurrah! However, I did feel excessive tension in my upper body after I was done. I thought that was strange, but since it wasn't my injured area, I assumed it was okay. I remember receiving a phone call from my Egoscue Method® therapist, John, shortly after finishing a run one day and commented to him about my upper body

tightness. He replied, "Why are you running with your upper body?"
Huh? I thought. I'm not. He explained that my body was searching
for stability, and since my pelvis wasn't solid and my hip muscles
were compensated, my search went all the way up the kinetic chain
to my upper back, neck and shoulders. And what better place? My
upper body was stiff as a board and dysfunctionally stable. Hmm . . .
I was starting to understand why. I gave up running for the time
being and instead focused on gaining the stability I needed in my
pelvis and the function I lacked in my hip muscles. Now that I teach
running technique and have greater awareness of body mechanics,
I can feel how overusing the upper body can take the load off of the
lower body and assist in propelling you forward. The body has an
amazing capacity for compensation!

So, instead of starting with complex multi-joint movements, which may
hide your compensations, corrective postural exercises isolate muscles and
make it very difficult to cheat. The smallest movements can seem harder
than an Olympic lift when you lack the coordination and strength in these
dysfunctional areas of your body. Simply
trying to turn on my left gluteal muscles made
me shake. These corrective posture exercises
often consist of isolating muscles through
static, isometric (same length) contractions
and slow, controlled movements of many repetitions. The body learns and grows stronger
through repeated practice. If you aren't able
to engage the muscles in a controlled setting,
it is highly unlikely you'll have access to
them under load when in motion.

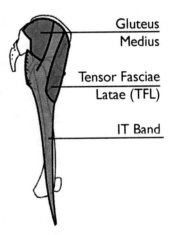

Gluteus
Medius

Tensor Fasciae
Latae (TFL)

IT Band

I've seen this happen with several young
female runners. These runners had developed a strong compensation pattern of using
their tensor fasciae latae (TFL) muscle for
the gluteus medius muscle (Figure 8-9).
Every time they went to run, they compensated, and their outer hips, where the TFL is
located, hurt.

Figure 8-9. The tensor
fasciae latae (TFL) muscle
often compensates for a weak
and dysfunctional gluteus
medius muscle.

body

The runners had tried different exercises in the weight room and changed their running strides, but their pain persisted. These women couldn't overcome their hip pain until compensated muscle patterns were changed and they learned to use their gluteus medius. This was accomplished through targeted corrective exercises.

When given a basic and small-scale exercise to isolate the gluteus medius, the runners had no sensation in their glutes. They could only feel their TFL engage. The runners had stopped using their gluteus medius and had lost connection with it. Their brain and glutes weren't talking anymore. Consequently, they had lost strength and function in the gluteus medius muscle, while their TFL grew stronger and stronger, overworking to the point of pain. With further manipulation of the exercise position to inhibit the TFL, along with more detailed exercise instructions, the runners finally started to feel their gluteus medius muscles working. Although their gluteus medius muscles were very weak, they were at least able to feel them enough to strengthen them.

Notice how specifically positioned and precise the movement had to be to engage the correct muscle. This is why standard weight training exercises didn't help; they allowed the runners to compensate. The movements were too complex and didn't force correct mechanics. Once strength was gained in the gluteus medius and the kinetic chain was functionally re-integrated, the athletes returned to running without pain.

A takeaway here is that the position of the body when performing an exercise is critical. It influences which muscles are activated. Remember, I couldn't do simple leg lifts in physical therapy. My problem was the position of my hip and pelvis and the orientation of the attached thigh muscles. While they were in their misaligned configuration, I could not engage the correct muscles to fire and lift my leg. Once I re-aligned my hip joint, and hence re-positioned my thigh muscles, I was successful. Mind you, this was not a mere twist of my hip in the pelvis. It took months of corrective posture exercises to achieve.

If muscle re-training is the missing piece to healing, where should you start? Answer: at the keystone of your posture—the pelvis—which was discussed in Chapter 6 and was also mentioned in relation to the gluteal muscles and the core in this chapter. This central pillar of body stability—the core—needs to be aligned and strengthened first, regardless of your symptoms, as you will read in the next chapter.

Summary

Postural deviations are the result of muscle imbalances, which lead to dysfunctions and compensations. Imbalanced muscles can be tight and short or tight and long, and both are weak. Two frequently experienced postural misalignments, rounding in the upper body and forward tilting of the pelvis, were discussed in this chapter. Tight hip flexors contribute to this deviated pelvic position, which can over-stretch the hamstrings and gluteal muscles. Improper length and tension in these muscles can lead to dysfunctions in these tissues and resultant compensations, such as when the gluteal muscles do not contract (dysfunction) and the lower back takes over the job of moving the leg behind the body (compensation).

Common approaches to correct the postural misalignments that have been caused by muscle imbalances include only passive repositioning modalities—massage, stretching, chiropractic—with short-lived results. In addition to repositioning, the body must be strengthened in good alignment and taught correct functional patterns of muscle engagement through re-training. Fundamental, isolated movements in precise positions are required to build strength without compensation. Once strength is gained, you, the athlete, can safely return to the multi-joint and complex movements that your sport requires without pain or increased risk of injury.

body

Game Winning Strategies

1. Obtain Optimal Hamstring Length and Pelvic Position

Hamstring length influences pelvic position. In this chapter I gave you one exercise to release your hip flexors—kneeling hip flexor stretch, and one exercise to shorten your hamstrings—hamstring and glute bridge. You can watch both exercises on my website. You'll find other examples on my blog.
Kneeling hip flexor stretch and hamstring and glute bridge videos: www.thepfathlete.com/resources
Find more pelvic positioning exercises: www.thepfathlete.com/blog

2. Attend a Posture Class

Inquire at your local health club, fitness center, YMCA, etc. about posture alignment class offerings.

3. Schedule a Posture Therapy Consultation or Appointment

Certified by Egoscue University®, I offer free consultations via phone or Skype.

To learn more about my posture therapy service visit:
www.thepfathlete.com/posture-therapy
or email me: jessica@thepfathlete.com

You can also search the Egoscue® website: www.egoscue.com to locate a local clinic or certified Egoscue Method® practitioner.

body

9

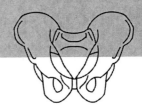

Starting With a Strong Core

*I*t's hard to build a good sandcastle. Sand is a slippery medium to work with and doesn't like to hold its structure. It inherently shifts and slides, leading to frequent cracks and complete collapses in sandcastle kingdoms, as shown in Figure 9-1. Beaches are littered with the remains of sand built fortresses. In sandcastle construction there are no rebar reinforcements or concrete footings. Not only is this building material soft and prone to fail, but there is no solid bedrock beneath.

Unlike the sandcastle, your body has a solid infrastructure: joint alignment. A balanced body is strong and able to perform the efficient, pain-free skills and movements needed for optimal sports performance. When your body lacks the solid infrastructure of aligned posture—the reinforcing rebar and bedrock that's missing in a sandcastle—your joints are not supported well. They slip around, like grains of sand in a sandcastle. However, instead of suffering a complete crash and being swept out to sea, your body remains upright. Stress cracks develop in the form of joint pain, muscle tightness, reduced flexibility, cartilage degeneration, and inflammation. These structural flaws can be observed as postural deviations, such as an elevated shoulder, a head tilt to one side, bowed or knocked knees, or turned-out feet, just to name a few. Through examining your posture in Chapter 7, you observed the state of your body's infrastructure. As a coach, I often have a client standing in front of me with several misalignments throughout their structure. Where do you start? *At the core!*

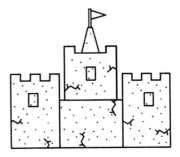

Figure 9-1. A sandcastle lacks a firm infrastructure.

Defining the Core

What is your core? And how does it relate to your posture? Although we hear a lot about "the core" and have been told we need a strong one from various sources—doctors, fitness professionals, media—there is still much confusion about what our core actually is. Why are we advised to strengthen our core for back pain? If we don't even know what the core is— if we don't know what we're trying to strengthen—how can we possibly train effectively?

For starters, the core is much more than just your abs. There continues to be a debate about what the core is. Many names have been applied and divisions made in reference to the core. In this discussion, I'm going to focus on only the essential structures of your core as they relate to posture. Simply put, your core is a cylinder of strength at the center of your body.[1] It is the deep infrastructure that you need to maintain alignment; it's the rebar and bedrock the sandcastle lacks that makes it prone to destruction.

Envision an apple core: it is round and fills the center of the apple in all directions. It is the solid framework around which the apple grows. Your core is no different. It is a cylinder of stability created by bones, muscles, and intra-abdominal pressure within your abdomen.[1] Just like an apple core that protects the fruit's precious seeds, your core cradles your life-sustaining organs, as shown in Figure 9-2.

The position of your core dictates the posture of your extremities—your arms, legs and head. Core alignment also influences the position of your internal organs, thus affecting the functioning of other body systems—digestion, respiration, circulation, elimination, etc. Your core radiates either strength and alignment or weakness and dysfunction throughout your body.

The main bony structures of your core are the rib cage, pelvis and spine—thoracic and lumbar. The rib cage and pelvis contain two of your

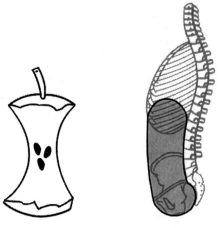

Figure 9-2. Your core resembles an apple core.

body's diaphragms. In the rib cage lies the respiratory diaphragm, and in the pelvis lies the pelvic diaphragm,[2] often referred to as the pelvic floor. I'll use the term "pelvic diaphragm" throughout this chapter. The respiratory diaphragm is one muscle, while the pelvic diaphragm is composed of several muscles together. The muscles of these diaphragms are skeletal muscles, just like your quadriceps or triceps, and they respond positively to training; they can also become weak from lack of use. *"Use it or lose it" applies to diaphragm muscles, too!*

The respiratory diaphragm forms the top of your core. The pelvic diaphragm forms the bottom. These diaphragm muscles extend laterally in all directions from your center—forward, backward, and to both sides—creating the caps of the cylindrical structure of your core. Spanning the space between the two diaphragms is the transverse abdominis (TA), the deepest abdominal muscle, which encircles the abdomen.[1] Figure 9-3 depicts the structures of the core. I often refer to the TA as your corset muscle. When it shortens, it compresses the center of the body inward, shrinking the waistline—*an additional reason to have a well-conditioned TA!* The multifidus muscle in the back is also often included as a core muscle, but I have chosen to exclude it for simplicity in this discussion.

The image of the core as shown in Figure 9-3 depicts the bones in correct alignment: the rib cage is centered above a level and neutrally positioned pelvis, and the spine has natural curves. This balanced core position is a big assumption, as it's usually incorrect for

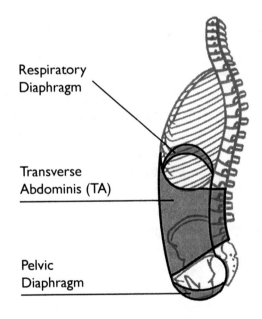

Respiratory Diaphragm

Transverse Abdominis (TA)

Pelvic Diaphragm

Figure 9-3. The bones (rib cage, pelvis, and spine) and the muscles (respiratory diaphragm, pelvic diaphragm and transverse abdominis) that make up the core.

body

175

many people. (Recall the pelvic asymmetry that was discussed in detail in Chapter 6.) For the purposes of defining the core, though, I took the liberty of depicting correct skeletal alignment.

Generating Internal Core Stability

The core muscles—respiratory diaphragm, pelvic diaphragm, and transverse abdominis (TA)—work together to generate internal stability. Since you are always breathing, your core is in continuous motion. Activation of your core happens in response to your breath. And the quality of your breath impacts how well your core functions. We'll get into that in Chapter 10; for now, let's focus on how internal stability is created.

According to Julie Wiebe, BSc, MPT, a women's sports medicine physical therapist and leader in pelvic floor education, your solid center is the result of two actions: one, a pressure increase in the abdominopelvic cavity that is created by the downward movement of the respiratory diaphragm on inhale—breathing air in—and two, an upward muscle contraction of the pelvic diaphragm and TA on exhale—breathing air out (Figure 9-4).[1]

Now that you have the big picture, let's break that down and talk first about your diaphragms. In a relaxed state, following exhalation, your respiratory and pelvic diaphragms, which create the top and bottom of your core respectively, should be in a lifted, domed-up position (though the pelvic diaphragm does not dome as high). I say "should be" because this is not always the case; issues with the diaphragm positions can lead to various forms of chronic pain. (You'll read more on this in Chapter 10) The larger respiratory diaphragm divides the thoracic cavity, which contains the lungs and heart, from the abdominopelvic cavity, which contains the multitude of our internal organs.[3] The pelvic diaphragm sits at the base of the abdominopelvic cavity. These diaphragms, placed on the opposite ends of your core, work together to create your internal stability.

When you inhale, both diaphragms move downward into a stretched position, as shown in Figure 9-5. The respiratory diaphragm descends into the abdominopelvic cavity. This reduces the pressure in the thoracic cavity and draws air into your lungs. The pelvic diaphragm also descends and lengthens, making room for all of your internal organs that have been pushed down.

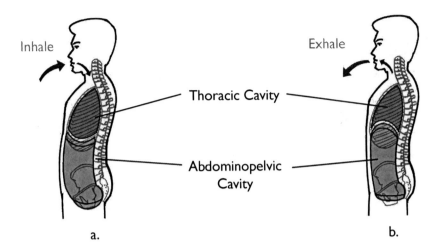

Inhale — Exhale

Thoracic Cavity

Abdominopelvic Cavity

a.

b.

Figure 9-4. The pressure in the core changes in response to the breath. (a) As the respiratory diaphragm moves down on inhalation, the pressure drops in the thoracic cavity and correspondingly increases in the abdominopelvic cavity. (b) The pressure gradient is reversed on exhale as the pelvic diaphragm and transverse abdominis contract.

body

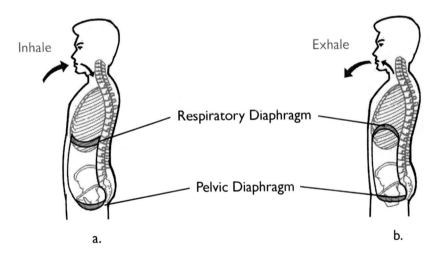

Inhale — Exhale

Respiratory Diaphragm

Pelvic Diaphragm

a.

b.

Figure 9-5. (a) During inhalation the respiratory and pelvic diaphragms descend and flatten. (b) During exhalation the diaphragms lift and dome up.

As pressure in the thoracic cavity goes down, there is a simultaneous increase in pressure in the abdominopelvic cavity. This increases your core stability. To maintain your core alignment—rib cage aligned over pelvis—while breathing in, your TA stretches and gently contracts to counter the forward expansion of the respiratory diaphragm (Figure 9-6[a]), which, if left unchecked, would lift your chest and flare your rib cage forward (Figure 9-6[b]).[2]

Upon exhale, the respiratory and pelvic diaphragms "should" (again, this doesn't always happen) ascend back up into a domed position, as shown in Figure 9-5. The core muscles, all in a lengthened position during inhale, now use the stored elastic energy that was created by the stretch of the muscles to recoil into a strong, contracted position. This adds further internal stability to your system.[1]

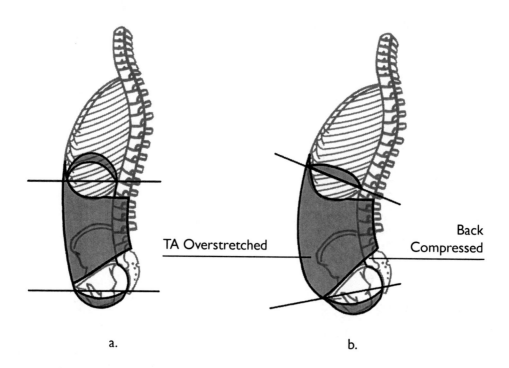

TA Overstretched

Back Compressed

a.

b.

Figure 9-6. (a) Aligned and (b) misaligned core breathing positions; improper breathing mechanics and overstretching of the transverse abdominis (TA) can result in an unbalanced and weak core.

Wiebe notes that pressure is an integral member of your core team—which also includes your three core muscles. Together, they create an ongoing cycle of stability. She compares this system to a piston moving up and down in your car. I also like the image of a slinky (Figure 9-7).

If you are not aligned in your core, you will not be able to transfer the pressure up and down the system. You will also not be able to move air, solids or fluids smoothly throughout your body. Your internal system's health is dependent on constant movement and flow.

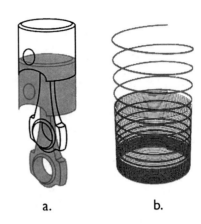

a.   b.

Figure 9-7. Your core oscillates up and down like a (a) piston or (b) slinky when you breathe.

The Problem With Belly Breathing

First of all, you don't have lungs in your belly, so the whole idea of air going into your stomach when breathing is wrong. In my experience, lying down, putting your hands on your belly and being instructed to "breathe into your belly" results in pushing the torso straight up toward the ceiling. Since we do not have lungs in our belly, it is not air that is causing the forward expansion of the belly. Postural adaptations are causing the action. All the core muscles are compromised in this breathing pattern. The unfortunate result of belly breathing is that the TA muscle overly lengthens, the rib cage flares up and out, the chest lifts, the pelvis tilts forward, the lower back extends—moving higher off the ground and thus causing compression—and the neck muscles tighten, as shown in Figure 9-6(b). Pushing the belly excessively forward upon inhale also changes the shape of the respiratory diaphragm, flattening it out, which reduces its effectiveness for proper respiration. This is what most people do when being told, "Belly breathe!" But it's obviously wrong. When you belly breathe, you lose your core alignment.

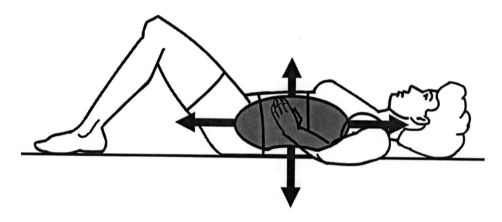

Figure 9-8. Breathe into your sides and back and throughout your torso while diaphragm breathing.

Instead of thinking "belly breathing," think "diaphragm breathing." Watch a video of this breathing technique on my website: www. thepfalthlete.com/resources.

Put your hands on the sides of your lower rib cage instead of on your belly when you breathe, as shown in Figure 9-8. When you inhale in this position, focus on expanding your torso backward and sideways, pushing the air outward into your hands and downward into the floor. There will also be some expansion forward, but really focus on moving the air backward and sideways, which is generally practiced less frequently. When breathing in this way, your abdominals don't over stretch. They maintain some tone. This abdominal resistance keeps the diaphragm in the correct position for efficient breathing without postural compensations. When done correctly, your chest and rib cage will expand, but not tilt upward. You'll feel your lower back lengthen and flatten into the ground instead of lifting up into further extension (or increased arch). When you diaphragm breathe in this way you maintain your core alignment and gain internal stability.

While you are learning to breathe from your diaphragm, I recommend focusing on breathing into one area at a time. For example, first try to feel your back flatten into the ground as you inhale. This front-to-back breathing pattern should be the most familiar, as you are probably accustomed to expanding your torso forward upon inhalation. Once you are having success with this, move on to expanding the air into your sides, and then from head to toe along your spine. You may find it more difficult to breathe into certain areas, and that's okay. Just keep practicing. Your body will respond. Once you can breathe into each area separately, combine them into a full breath that expands in all directions. And don't forget about your posture on the exhale! Be mindful that you are also maintaining a good position as the air exits your body.

What About Kegels?

First, for those who don't know, a Kegel is an exercise to help strengthen the pelvic diaphragm. Introduced in 1948 by Dr. Arnold Henry Kegel, a gynecologist, this movement continues to be a primary exercise prescribed for pelvic floor incontinence (leaking urine).[4] Urinary incontinence most often occurs in response to any stressor that creates a sudden and dramatic change in internal pressure, such as coughing, jumping, sneezing, heavy lifting, and running. The Kegel is performed by contracting the muscles that stop urination; by holding for a few seconds; and then by relaxing and repeating. There are three fundamental reasons why I am not an advocate of Kegels.

My primary criticism of the Kegel exercise is that it does not address alignment before strengthening. As you've read, a strong core starts with good alignment. But what if the pelvis itself, to which the pelvic diaphragm muscles attach, is out of position? What if the pelvic diaphragm muscles are asymmetrical—some are lengthened and some are shortened, as shown in Figure 9-9? Do you want to strengthen the pelvic diaphragm muscles in this orientation? Can you even do it? Probably not. Performing a Kegel under these circumstances is likely going to exacerbate your problem.

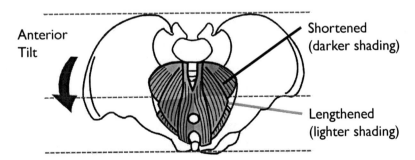

Anterior Tilt

Shortened (darker shading)

Lengthened (lighter shading)

Figure 9-9. The pelvic diaphragm muscles are asymmetrical and weak when the pelvic bones are misaligned.

body

This is why integrating the breath into core exercises is so important! Pressure is distributed throughout the body as a response to the breath; this change in pressure in the core is disbursed to other areas. If you look closely at the core—and beyond—in Figure 9-10, you'll see there are many open spaces within the skeleton of the body through which pressure changes can be directed.[5]

Notice the large hole in the center of the pelvis and the two smaller ones within each of the left and right hip bones. The rib cage is also a large, open cavity. And, within the skull there are many openings, including a hole at the base of the skull, eye sockets, nose passageways, and space on either side of the jaw. When pressure is distributed into these open spaces in response to breathing, the surrounding bones move.[5] Figure 9-11 demonstrates how the ribs move out and in as the intra-abdominal pressures changes with inhalation, 9-11(a) and exhalation, 9-11(b).

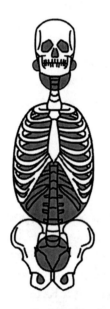

Figure 9-11 demonstrates the movement: just as the ribs move out and in as the intra-abdominal pressure changes with breathing, so do the bones around these open cavities.[5]

Most relevant to our present discussion of Kegels is the response of the pelvic bones to the pressure changes that are created by the breath. Basically, the bones of your pelvis move and change position when you breathe, like the ribs. You can think of your pelvic bones as having a position of inspiration and expiration, just as the ribs have a position of inspiration and expiration, as shown in Figure 9-11. I know, I'm getting pretty technical again, so I am going to skip the specific postural changes in the pelvic bones with breathing. All you need to remember is that by using the proper sequencing of breathing during your core training, you can reposition your pelvis—and, correspondingly, the pelvic diaphragm—at the same time.

Figure 9-10. The body has several open cavities, as depicted by the gray areas in this image, that expand and contract with the breath.

In some cases, pelvic asymmetry is causing the pelvic diaphragm to be weak because the musculature is in a poor position. When the pelvis returns to a neutral position, the pelvic diaphragm muscles return to their correct length and tension, where they are strong. The first step, then, toward a stronger pelvic diaphragm is balancing the pelvis. Kegels certainly won't correct pelvic orientation.

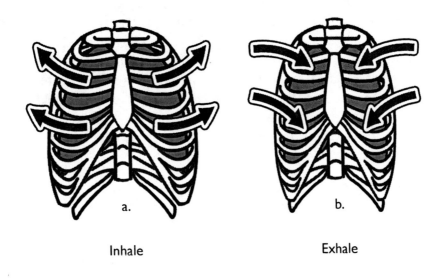

a.   b.

Inhale   Exhale

Figure 9-11. (a) The ribs move outward as the pressure decreases in the thoracic cavity and the lungs fill with air during inhalation. (b) The ribs move inward as the pressure increases in the thoracic cavity and the lungs are emptied of air during exhalation.

Julie Wiebe points out the second problem with this exercise: "Kegels have only taught your pelvic floor [diaphragm] to hold. This does not teach it to be responsive to the changing pressure in the abdomen."[1] All of the stress-inducing activities listed previously—sneezing, jumping, etc.—involve large pressure changes in the abdomen. These large pressure changes can easily overwhelm a pelvic diaphragm that only knows how to hold. The pelvic diaphragm needs to be able to go up and down, like a piston or slinky (Figure 9-7). It needs to be adaptable and able to respond to pressure changes. As Wiebe says, your pelvic diaphragm needs to "bounce." Kegels can produce a hypertonic (too much tension) pelvic diaphragm. This makes it very hard for these muscles to move up and down smoothly, which is needed to create internal stability during rapid pressure fluctuations.

Finally, Kegels are typically done in isolation of the other core muscles. Wiebe emphasizes that the pelvic diaphragm needs to be trained to work simultaneously with the other core muscles. She refers to the three core muscles—respiratory diaphragm, pelvic diaphragm and transverse abdominis (TA)—as gears that cannot turn without all the gears in place. I love her statement about the continuous oscillation of the core "moving at the rhythm of the diaphragm."[6] I like to think of the respiratory diaphragm as the motor of your core machine. The pelvic diaphragm, which responds to the movement of the respiratory diaphragm, needs to learn how to coordinate with the other muscles on exhale, particularly with the abdominals. Kegels do not integrate the muscles and function of the core.

Just say no to Kegels and yes to an aligned pelvis with co-activation of the core muscles synchronized with your breath!

Weakness in the Core

When we think about issues such as stress-incontinence, or, as you've learned, leaking urine in response to pressure changes in the core system, we generally picture a mom who has had several children, is advancing in years, and carries a few extra pounds. Well, throw that image away—*right now!* I was an athlete in my teens when I had this humiliating problem. This is not something I generally talk about, but it is pertinent to the discussion. My core had been dysfunctional for a long time, although I didn't know it. I only spoke of this problem once as a teenager. I didn't mention it again until many years later.

As a young gymnast, I struggled with urinary leakage due to the stress produced in my pelvic diaphragm during high velocity tumbling and landings. It was embarrassing and demeaning, not to mention quite a difficult issue to deal with during competition. No one ever spoke of such problems on my team, and I felt very alone. When my coach noticed my predicament, she was of no help. She only made me feel worse by ridiculing me and my situation. I was scared and thought there must be something really wrong with me. Of course, there was, but not in the way I imagined.

You would think that out of all athletes, a gymnast who has had hours of "core" training would be strong. Not so! Do you think this set me up for my later surgeries and dysfunctions? I'd bet on it!

Incontinence, often kept as a private and secret issue by clients, has a dramatic impact on sports and quality of life, as my client Maurine explains:

> Running was my first love, and I've been a runner for as long as I can remember. In my earlier years my life revolved around running events and each goal that I set for myself: 5ks, 10ks, half-marathons, marathons, triathlons, and more. Unfortunately, as I got older, running and other exertional activities came with a price—incontinence. By the time I was in my late 30's, it was becoming increasingly problematic. I found myself purposefully dehydrating myself before events. Lack of proper hydration lead to periodic migraines and, at one point, heat stroke after a triathlon event. Then I developed a uterine fibroid. My OBGYN physician thought perhaps the fibroid was pushing on my bladder, so I had a hysterectomy in the hopes that this would remedy the embarrassing incontinence problem. It didn't. To learn how to strengthen the perineal [pelvic diaphragm] muscles, she sent me to a physical therapist who specialized in biofeedback therapy. I traveled two hours each way to those appointments. I did many daily Kegel exercises. In the end, they proved futile. I wondered why I was having this issue, particularly since I'd never given birth! Since then I've been fortunate enough to discover that, all along, the real source of the issue was an extended pelvis or lordosis [increased arch in the back], which causes the perineal muscles to be stretched. When stretched, those muscles can't fire. The only thing that has significantly helped is postural alignment therapy.

body

As a society, we are reluctant to talk about these kinds of sensitive issues, choosing to ignore them, hoping they will just go away. Well, I can attest that these problems only get worse with time and age. *The pelvic diaphragm is simply a group of muscles.* So, why can't we talk about it? I suppose it's because of its close proximity to the sexual organs, which we never refer to directly or indirectly. Seriously? Are we really that prudish?

Have you watched TV lately? *This is a matter of health!* Many people are not diagnosed correctly because of our Puritan approach. The pelvis is the keystone of our posture, and yet the pelvic diaphragm muscles sit within its structure—forgotten.

Strengthening the Core

Your core is a strong, solid center that supports your posture. It is deep within your body. The more this internal stability is lost, the more the surface muscles are called upon to take on an increased postural support role. In addition, the core muscles themselves, primarily the respiratory diaphragm, might also take on a postural role, which I'll discuss in Chapter 10.

Your trunk consists of many layers of muscles, as shown in Figure 9-12. The most superficial ones, like the rectus abdominis ("six-pack muscle") and paraspinal muscles on your back, lie just under the skin.

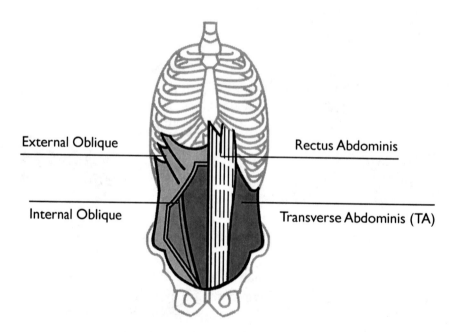

External Oblique

Rectus Abdominis

Internal Oblique

Transverse Abdominis (TA)

Figure 9-12. Your core muscles lie at the deepest position within your trunk. The shading in the image indicates depth. The TA is shaded the darkest and is deepest within the core.

Without a solid core, the more external muscles become primary in posture. In my case, they were nearly all that was holding me up. No wonder my back couldn't shut off; *no wonder it always hurt!* These muscles couldn't stop working if I were to stay upright. My disabling lower back pain was not from a lack of strength in my superficial abdominals or lower back. Rather, these muscles were overly developed and doing all of the work. Muscle imbalance and dysfunction happens from the inside out.[7] The core goes first, and the outer muscles compensate. I challenge you to consider extremely toned abdominals as a possible sign that they are overworking at the expense of the deeper stabilizing core muscles.

If core strength starts with alignment as I've discussed, then core strengthening exercises should be performed in an attempt to fortify a neutral position of the core bones—rib cage, pelvis, spine—and the supporting muscles and soft tissue. This training begins with awareness. With private clients and in my classes, one of the first things I often do is provide education about core alignment—rib cage positioned directly over pelvis. If you think of your rib cage as a bell, you want the clapper (the part that rings the bell) hanging straight down through the center of the pelvis,[8] as shown in Figure 9-13(a).

When the rib cage is positioned correctly over the pelvis, the spine is aligned with its natural curves, and the head is balanced on top. To experience this position, I have my clients or class members turn sideways to the mirror and notice their posture. Often they'll see a lifted rib cage with the chest and breasts angling upwards and an accentuated curve in the low back. Their rib cage bell is rung up and forward, as shown in Figure 9-13(b).

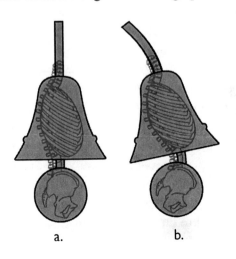

a.   b.

Figure 9-13. (a) When the core is aligned, the rib cage bell is positioned directly over the pelvis. (b) When the core is misaligned, the rib cage bell is rung up, the pelvis tilts too far forward, and the lower back is overly arched.

body

Most of us have all been taught to stand up straight by pulling our shoulders back. However, we frequently tend to overdo it. Upon observing our side posture, we notice that we have pulled our shoulders too far back so that they are positioned behind our hips, with rib cage and chest lifted. If this sounds familiar, you're right. This was my posture (Figure 8-2). In this position, there is too much length through the front of the body and not enough length in the back of the body, particularly the low back. In this posture, the lower back is being compressed and often hurts. Notice how I just described the misaligned breathing position shown in Figure 9-6(b). Breathing patterns, posture, and pain are frequently connected. Stay tuned for more on this in Chapter 10.

To alleviate this often-painful state of the lower back being compressed, the muscles in the front of the body need to shorten and the back muscles need to lengthen. This is accomplished by drawing the rib cage down, back and in. To do this, move the bottom of your rib cage down toward your pelvis, back toward your spine and in toward your center. Essentially, you are changing your posture from the misaligned position shown in Figure 9-13(b) to the aligned position shown in Figure 9-13(a). Often this adjustment alone will alleviate back pain symptoms. When your core is aligned, your structure is supported by your bones as it should be; it's not solely being held up by your superficial muscles.

If you felt your shoulders move forward when you modified your posture to align your core, that's okay. You are supposed to have a slight rounding in your mid-upper back. You may, however, have some tightness through your tissues in the front of your chest, shoulder and neck that needs to be released in order to allow the shoulders to come back into a neutral position. In many of the activities we perform in daily life—using electronic devices, cooking, driving, writing, etc.—our hands are in front of our bodies, shortening and tightening these tissues. Additional repositioning of your shoulder blades might also be necessary to achieve good upper body posture. Nevertheless, this is the position you need to attain with your core—rib cage over pelvis— to be strong.

This simple adjustment is something you can do several times a day, whenever you think about it. The more you position your core in good alignment, the stronger you are becoming in this position, and the easier it will be for you to hold. Although it may feel strange now, this improved position will eventually feel natural. A client going through posture therapy commented to me that his body had adapted so well to the new, aligned posture that he now hurts when he finds himself in his old, slouched position, which used to relieve his pain. The body can change, and quite quickly, with consistent reminders.

Gaining core alignment is the first step toward greater strength. Any further resistance exercises, from chest presses to step-ups, need to be done with an aligned core. When that's the case, you're building your core strength and alignment with every exercise you do. *Cool!* Of course, you can do exercises that target the core directly. One of my favorites is the pelvic tilt.

Practice Pelvic Tilt Exercises

You can watch a video of this exercise on my website: www.thepfathlete.com/resources.

1. Lie on the ground with your knees bent at 90 degrees and your upper body relaxed, arms out to your sides with your palms up.

2. Maintain sensory awareness of your heels and big toes without pushing into the ground for proper alignment of the feet, knees, and hips. There is a tendency for the feet to roll out, which is why you need to keep the big toes down. This is best felt with bare feet.

3. Start the movement by tilting your pelvis gently up toward your head so that your lower back lengthens and flattens into the ground while your rib cage rotates down in front (anterior). Your lower anterior ribs will come closer to the front of your pelvis. Simultaneously, your posterior rib cage rotates up and backward, so that your upper back ribs move closer to your scapulae and press harder into the floor just below your shoulder blades, as shown in Figure 9-14. Watch that your shoulders do not round forward. As you tilt your pelvis, push your knees forward slightly to engage your deep transverse abdominis (TA) muscle. Avoid over-contracting your rectus abdominis ("six-pack muscle"). Keep this muscle relaxed.

body

189

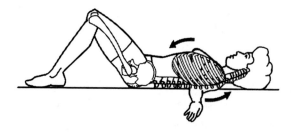

Figure 9-14. The rib cage rotates to flatten the lower back.

4. Next, tilt your pelvis forward toward your heels. Your lower back will lift off the ground into an arch, as shown in Figure 9-15(b).

   NOTE: The movement of the pelvis during this exercise is accomplished by using the surrounding muscles—abdominals, back and hips—and not by simply lifting and lowering your lumbar spine. Strive to feel the different muscles engage as you tilt your pelvis back and forth.

5. Coordinate the movement with your breathing: exhale out through your mouth as you flatten your back (Figure 9-15[a]), and inhale through your nose as you arch your back (Figure 9-15[b]). You'll feel your TA and oblique abdominals engage to pull your ribs down, back and in as you exhale and flatten your back to the floor. One of the under-appreciated but essential roles of your abdominals is forced exhalation. *Your abdominals are exhalation muscles!*

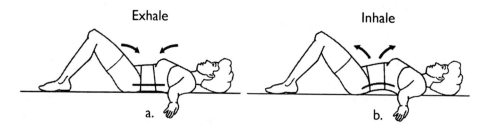

Exhale   Inhale

a.   b.

Figure 9-15. Pelvic tilts strengthen the core musculature by integrating the breath.

NOTE: Inhaling through your nose with your lips touching and tongue on the top of your mouth facilitates correct head, jaw and neck posture without over activating the neck muscles. Exhaling out your mouth during the exercise enhances contraction of the core muscles.

6. Integrate the pelvic diaphragm muscles into this exercise by pulling up gently with these muscles (similar to what you would do as though you were stopping the flow of urine) as you exhale. Become aware of the natural movement of your pelvic diaphragm in response to your breath on inhale—moving down and lengthening—and exhale—lifting and shortening.

7. Hold the exhaled/back flat position for three seconds before moving into the arch.

8. Repeat this exercise 10-30 times.

Your Core Foundation

I began this chapter talking about sandcastles. Hopefully, this analogy to your body makes more sense now, and you have a greater appreciation for your core. Julie Wiebe aptly describes how your core acts as an anchor, or foundation, for movement.[1] It provides stability for all of the other muscles to pull against when you move. To move without compensation, the core must activate first. She tells her clients to "blow before you go"[1] to activate the core before moving. This is why you are usually cued to exhale on the exertion portion of a weight lift. I'll talk more about how to integrate core strength and breathing into your resistance training in Chapter 12. Before I go on to that topic, however, I'm going to devote the next chapter to the second role of your respiratory diaphragm: *breathing!* How you breathe greatly impacts your alignment, motion, and chronic pain.

Summary

Your core provides the foundation for your structure. A strong core facilitates symmetrical posture and uncompensated, pain-free movement. Core strength starts with core alignment: the rib cage positioned directly over a balanced pelvis and the spine in its natural curves. The fundamental muscles of the core are the respiratory and pelvic diaphragms and the transverse abdominis (TA). These muscles work together like gears to create a cylinder of stability in your center through integration of pressure and muscle contraction. The pressure generated by the breath causes bones to move, creating postures of inhalation and exhalation. The body needs to be able to transition smoothly between these positions.

The core is in constant motion, moving up and down within your torso (like a piston or slinky) in time with your breathing. If your core is not aligned, this oscillation within your center cannot happen, which leads to weakness and stagnation throughout your body systems. Belly breathing compromises core alignment. Diaphragm breathing with torso expansion in all directions upon inhale should be practiced instead.

Urinary incontinence results from a weak core that cannot respond to rapid pressure changes. There are several flaws in the Kegel exercise—strengthening before alignment, focusing solely on holding, and contracting the pelvic diaphragm muscles in isolation. The core muscles lie at the deepest level within the abdomen. They need to be strengthened in unison through small movements, like the pelvic tilt exercise. The core should engage before movement. An aligned and strong core is essential to reduce chronic pain and injury risk so that you can play for the long term.

Game Winning Strategies

1. Increase Your Core Awareness

Is your rib cage bell positioned directly on top of your pelvis? Find a mirror and take a look. Really feel your position when your core is aligned. *When you adjust your posture in this way, what changes within your body?* Find some form of physical feedback, such as a sensation in your body—how your weight is distributed in your feet, for instance—that can help you recognize when you are in a good core position versus a poor core position. Then check in with your body often. Notice your core alignment when you are walking, stretching, folding clothes, brushing your teeth, sitting at your computer . . . You get the idea. Check in often.

2. Become Aware of How You Breathe

Do you belly breathe? This can compromise your alignment and increase your pain with each breath. Practice diaphragm breathing as discussed in this chapter and as shown on my website:
www.thepfathlete.com/resources.

3. Strengthen Your Core

In this chapter I gave you one example of a core strengthening exercise, the pelvic tilt, which you can watch on my website. However, there are many more exercises to tone your core. You'll find other examples on my blog. Whatever exercise you choose, just remember the fundamentals: keep your core aligned, activate all of your core muscles together, and synchronize your breathing.
Pelvic tilt video: www.thepfathlete.com/resources
Find more core exercises: www.thepfathlete.com/blog

body

10

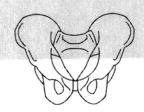

Breathing Yourself Into Balance

"You don't breathe well." This was the first thing that John, my Egoscue Method® posture therapist, said to me during my initial postural assessment. *Huh?* I had no idea what he was talking about. It didn't make any sense. *What in the world could breathing have to do with my back and hip pain?* Since he didn't say any more about it, I let it go.

But the idea of my faulty breathing being connected to my chronic pain wouldn't go away. A couple of years following that posture assessment, my structural integration therapist Sonia noticed that I couldn't get much air into the back of my lungs. *You're supposed to be able to breathe into your back?* She explained how the lungs sit in the middle of your torso and can expand front to back, side to side, and up and down, as shown in Figure 10-1. That was a new idea for me.

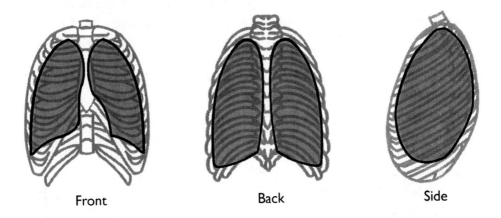

Front   Back   Side

Figure 10-1. The lungs fill the space within the rib cage in all directions.

My respiratory diaphragm, the primary muscle of inspiration, wasn't moving well. When a breathing coach put his hands on my back at the level of my diaphragm, he could barely sense any movement. My diaphragm was stuck. As I mentioned in the last chapter, your core muscles can become postural muscles. In my case, my diaphragm was working as a postural stabilizer,[1] holding a rigid position. Instead of helping me breathe, my diaphragm was trying to provide the infrastructure I lacked because my core was stiff and weak. A supple core is a strong core, and mine was definitely not supple.

With little involvement from my respiratory diaphragm, nearly all of my breathing occurred in my upper lungs and chest. The extent of my faulty breathing mechanics became distressingly clear while taking a course, *Myokinematic Restoration*, hosted by the Postural Restoration Institute® (PRI).[2] When I tried to blow up a balloon using proper muscle engagement of my diaphragm and intercostal muscles, I felt like my neck muscles were going to spasm and might burst from under my skin. Since I didn't know how to breathe effectively with my diaphragm, I had learned to rely on my accessory muscles for respiration—neck, back, shoulder and chest muscles.[3]

The Posture—Breath Connection

So, I couldn't breathe well. Instead, I used my accessory muscles to move air in and out of my body. That didn't seem like a big deal to me. It might hinder my athletic pursuits because I wasn't using my full lung capacity, but past that, *what does it really matter?* Well, for starters, it meant that my core was dysfunctional. Additionally, it meant that I was compensating and causing strain within my body when I moved. That's not good. Poor breathing also meant that I was going to have a hard time changing my posture because I was reinforcing my asymmetrical position approximately 20,000 times a day,[4] the average number of breaths a person takes in 24 hours.

Breathing keeps us alive; it is imperative to our survival. This basic need is going to supersede nearly every other physiological function. It is certainly going to override postural symmetry. The body will figure out a way to create the space and pressure gradient needed to bring air into our lungs. It will cheat any way necessary to accomplish this task. If air doesn't get in, we die. If our bones get twisted around and our tissues become misaligned in the process, so be it. I'd rather be crooked and in pain than dead. *Breath truly is life!*

When I breathed with my accessory respiratory muscles—neck, back, shoulder and chest muscles—I put my body into a position of extension, as shown in Figure 10-2(a). My lower back became more arched; my rib cage moved up and out, away from the spine, which impacted the position of my shoulders; my pelvis tilted too far forward; and my neck stretched out, giving me a forward head posture. Let's contrast my extended posture with the image of optimal posture, as shown in Figure 10-2(b), focusing first on the position of the respiratory diaphragm.

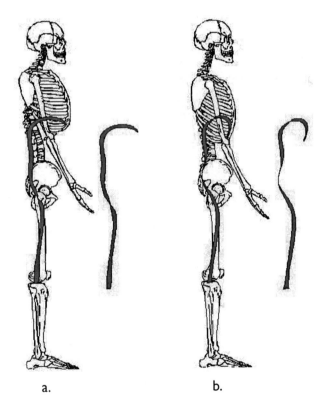

a.   b.

Figure 10-2. (a) Extended posture and (b) optimal posture, shown with the line of the Anterior Interior Chain (AIC) of muscles within and in front of the skeletons.

Figure used with permission from the Postural Restoration Institute® © 2016, *Postural Respiration Manual*, www.posturalrestoration.com.

In Chapter 9, I referred to the respiratory diaphragm as the motor of your core machine. This diaphragm also drives posture. When comparing the images in Figure 10-2, notice the difference in the position of the respiratory diaphragm, which is the top part of the line sitting within the rib cage. The respiratory diaphragm is at the top of the Anterior Interior Chain (AIC) of muscles that extends down to the side of the knee. It is drawn as a line on and in front of the images in Figure 10-2. This is a chain of muscles that works together as a unit. As I described in Chapter 5, the body moves through integrated kinetic chains. The AIC consists of the respiratory diaphragm, psoas, iliacus, tensor fasciae latae (TFL), vastus lateralis and biceps femoris.[2] Primarily, the AIC includes your diaphragm, hip flexors, and lateral quadricep and hamstring.

In optimal posture, Figure 10-2(b), the respiratory diaphragm is domed: a relaxed position. However, in extended posture, Figure 10-2(a), it is stretched out: a tense position. Observe, too, that this change in the respiratory diaphragm also affects rib cage position. As the respiratory diaphragm flattens, the rib cage flares up and forward.

Now let's consider how poor breathing affects the other end of the core, at the level of the pelvic diaphragm. Although not as easy to see, the pelvis tilts forward in extended posture. As we struggle to bring air into our bodies when in extended posture, we use our accessory muscles: the neck, back, shoulder and chest muscles. To expand the front of our bodies, we lift our chest using our neck and shoulders and arch our lower backs, which facilitates a forward tilt of the pelvis. If you look closely at Figures 10-2(a) and (b), you'll notice that the tailbone, at the base of the sacrum, protrudes back and out more in (a) than in (b). Following from this, you might also observe that the top of the hip bone is tilted more forward in (a) than (b). This forward tilt of the pelvis changes the length and tension in the pelvic diaphragm muscles. Like the respiratory diaphragm, the pelvic diaphragm is in an overly stretched, tight, and weak position.

Remember the caveat I made in the previous chapter about how the respiratory and pelvic diaphragms "should", but do not always, ascend back up into a relaxed position on exhale? Well, this is what I was referring to. Neither of these diaphragms can ascend when the body is in extended posture. Diaphragms either work together, or they fail together. They both move up and down like the two ends of a piston, or they both become stretched and inflexible.

Another postural deviation that happens in response to the forward tilting of the pelvis in extended posture is repositioning of the leg bone (femur). In Chapter 6, I discussed the relationship between hip and knee position. Essentially, the hip and knee are opposite ends of the same bone, the femur, and they move in the same direction. However, what influences femur position is the pelvis. When the hip bone has too much anterior tilt, the acetabulum (hip socket) moves down and forward, and the femur follows, frequently positioning itself inward,[5] as shown in Figure 10-3.

Poor breathing, then, contributed to the torsion in my knees, which led to three left knee surgeries and an eventual left hip surgery. Poor breathing also increased the arch in my lower back, contributing to my unrelenting back pain, as I'll discuss shortly. And that's only the lower body! *I guess correct breathing is a big deal!*

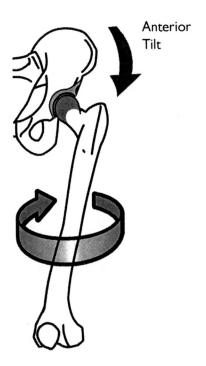

Anterior Tilt

Figure 10-3. When the hip bone increases its anterior tilt, the femur often becomes directed inward.[5]

body

Posture Displays Breathing Patterns

My extended posture reflected my pattern of breathing—mainly into my chest and using my accessory respiratory muscles. How, you want to know? Thanks for asking! Let me explain.

Review the breathing mechanics information from Chapter 9: upon inhalation, the respiratory and pelvic diaphragms move down, lengthen and flatten; upon exhalation, the diaphragms "should" move back up into relaxed domed positions. My respiratory and pelvic diaphragms were stuck in a lengthened and flattened position. This is a position of inhalation. Check it out for yourself. Take a deep breath in and hold it for 10 seconds. Now notice your posture. If you're like most athletes, you ended up in a position of extension, ranging from mild to severe, like Figure 10-2(a). If this is how your body has adapted to get air into your lungs, you will repeat this pattern thousands of times a day, regardless of your activity.

Now let's try the opposite: exhale all of your air out and hold for 10 seconds. What happened to your posture? Hopefully, your ribs came down and you looked more like the optimal posture image in Figure 10-2(b). Did you notice a difference in the difficulty of holding either position? I find it much harder to hold my breath after exhaling, not just physically but also cognitively. When I first did this exercise at *Pelvis Restoration,* a course hosted by the Postural Restoration Institute® (PRI),[1] I became anxious and a little scared; it was a fight not to give up early and take in more air. Not too surprising, I guess, since exhaling is the last thing we'll do in this life. Then, when I did take a breath in, after pausing after a full exhale, it was a big breath. I didn't feel this desperate need for air when holding my breath after an inhale. How about you? Are you as comfortable in a posture of inspiration as expiration? I realize there may be some physiological factors contributing here, but I still find it interesting.

When you are not able to exhale completely, excess air remains in your lungs, making your next inhale less effective and negatively affecting your posture. James, my instructor in the *Myokinematic Restoration* course, observed that this trapped air was like having a beach ball stuck in your torso. With this mass of air in your center, it is difficult to attain optimal posture by bringing the ribs down in front over this obstruction. However, complete exhalation is necessary to obtain optimal posture. To change my posture and reach this ideal, I needed to learn how to exhale. Do you need to improve your ability to remove air from your body as I did? *It's possible!* I can now do this exhalation exercise with much greater ease.

How did I get stuck in an extended, inhalation posture? Sports may be partly to blame. When breathing hard and exerting yourself, taking in air becomes one of your fundamental concerns. You need to get air in to keep going. Pushing air out seems of less importance. Have you noticed that after an all-out sprint, athletes will bend forward, putting their hands on their knees to help them regain their breath? I believe this is to improve diaphragm position, which promotes breathing efficiency and better exhalation. Improper breathing is also a leading cause of side stitches with runners. Advice to reduce these annoying cramps often involves breathing mechanics, specifically exhaling.[6]

As athletes, we like a hard workout. We crave movement. We need to feel the burn of an intense effort. Being still and breathing is often the most difficult thing I ask of my clients. It's a different kind of exercise. Instead of grinding out another exhausting interval where your heart is pounding through your chest, you have to be still, inwardly focused, and notice the subtleties of how your body accomplishes the task of breathing.

I couldn't believe what a workout it was to breathe correctly. *I broke a sweat!* My abdominals, which I had previously thought to be strong, actually quivered as I held them tight to keep my rib cage down after exhaling. *Unbelievable!*

Lumbar Extension: Tight Hip Flexors or Flat Diaphragm?

My extended posture caused debilitating back pain. As you can see in the image of extended posture in Figure 10-2(a), the lumbar spine is overly arched. If you lie down on your back on a hard surface with your knees bent, you'll probably notice space between your lower back and the floor. Go ahead, do it now. I'll be here when you get back.

Some space between your lower back and the floor is normal. The lumbar spine is supposed to have an arch. If, however, the arch in your lumbar spine is high off the ground like mine was, you might wonder what is causing this excessive arch in your back. There are two potential causes for this: first, tight hip flexors, or second, a flat diaphragm.

Through the Egoscue Method®, I learned that this arch is caused by tight hip flexors—the psoas and iliacus—which are the muscles located on the front of your hip,[7] as shown in Figure 10-4.

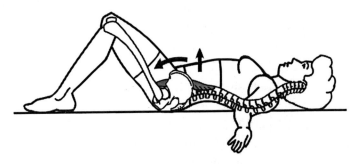

Figure 10-4. The pelvis is pulled forward by short and tight hip flexor muscles, creating a lumbar arch.

Through the Postural Restoration Institute® (PRI), I learned that this arch is caused by a flattened diaphragm and poor breathing. When the diaphragm lengthens, the rib cage moves away from the spine and pulls the lower back with it into an arch,[1] as shown in Figure 10-5.

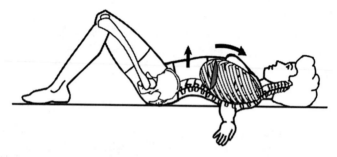

Figure 10-5. The pelvis is pulled forward by a flared rib cage and flattened diaphragm, creating a lumbar arch.

Which is right? Actually, both are correct. The hip flexors and diaphragm are intricately linked through connective tissue and are part of the Anterior Interior Chain (AIC) discussed previously. Many attempts have been made to separate these muscles through dissection, without success.[1] The psoas muscle, your primary hip flexor, is the only muscle to connect the upper and lower body. The muscle itself runs from the inner femur (the lesser trochanter for the anatomically inclined) to all five lumbar vertebrae and the twelfth thoracic vertebrae and intervertebral discs.[3] The diaphragm is a large muscle encircling your abdomen, spreading forward to your sternum, sideways to the ribs, and backward and down to the lumbar spine.[3] *Aha!* The psoas and diaphragm both have attachments to the lumbar spine, as shown in Figure 10-6.

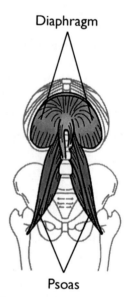

Diaphragm

Psoas

Figure 10-6. The psoas and diaphragm are joined through unyielding soft tissue connections at the lumbar spine.

Tom Myers, acclaimed fascia expert, explains it well: "The diaphragm is rooted to the lower body through the leg."[8] Looking at Figure 10-6, it becomes more apparent that changes in the position of the diaphragm, and therefore faulty breathing, can affect pelvic, back, hip and femur position, and vice-versa. Correcting my exaggerated lumbar arch required not only lengthening my hip flexors but also learning how to breathe correctly so that my diaphragm could relax into a domed position. In treatment, the entire chain needs to be considered, not just one end. When I personally practiced and taught Egoscue Method® E-cises™ to my students and clients, I was mainly focused on releasing the tension in the hip flexors. Aside from telling my clients to breathe, I didn't give any consideration to the position of the diaphragm or how it might be affecting posture. Now that we know better, instead of just stretching hip flexors like crazy, we'll integrate breathing and correct diaphragm position into our routines. By doing so, we'll improve our core alignment. *Bonus!*

Return of the Overly Lengthened Hamstrings

As you have just read, the hip flexors and respiratory diaphragm are integrated muscles, and together, they affect pelvic position and lumbar extension. The shortened hip flexors and lengthened respiratory diaphragm pull the pelvis forward, creating an anterior tilt and subsequent arch in the lower back. The question to ask now is this: which muscles pull the pelvis backward to reduce the exaggerated arch? I mentioned this briefly in Chapter 8, but if you don't remember, the title of this section gives you the answer: *Hamstrings!* Please appreciate that there are additional muscles, including the abdominals (which have been discussed previously), that contribute to pelvic position, some of which are shown in Figure 10-7. However, for simplicity in making my point, I will limit my discussion to the hip flexors and hamstrings.

If you refer back to the image of optimal posture, Figure 10-2(b), you'll observe that the line drawn within and in front of the figure, the AIC, does not end with the hip flexor attachment on the upper leg bone. It continues down the leg to the side of the knee. As I mentioned in Chapter 1, the fundamental goal of Postural Restoration® is maintaining proper diaphragm positions. In this case, we are referring to the respiratory and pelvic diaphragms.

body

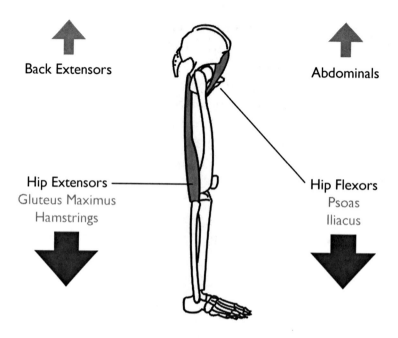

Figure 10-7. The hamstrings and hip flexors, along with other muscles,[3] exert opposing forces on the pelvis to keep it in a balanced position.

The muscles down the leg, the lower part of the AIC, primarily the biceps femoris (hamstring muscle), assists in keeping the pelvis and diaphragms in neutral positions. The hamstrings pull the pelvis from behind and don't allow it to tilt too far forward,[9] thereby inhibiting extended posture (Figure 10-2[a]), facilitating neutral posture (Figure 10-2[b]), and maintaining proper diaphragm positions.

However, all bets are off when the hamstrings are overly lengthened and dysfunctional. When in this long and weak position, the hamstrings cannot adequately oppose the forward pull of the hip flexors. As a result, the body goes into an extended posture (Figure 10-2[a]), and proper diaphragm positions, as well as efficient breathing mechanics and optimal posture, are lost.

Two Hemidiaphragms and a Twist in Your Rib Cage

Okay, enough with the diaphragms, already. I know, you get it: breathing and diaphragm positions are important. They impact other joints and chronic pain. You understand this vital concept, but there's more you need to know. The truth is, I've been holding out on you. Not because I'm mean, but because I wanted to present one concept at a time to make the information easier to absorb. So here's the deal. Up to this point, for simplicity's sake, I've presented the respiratory diaphragm as one big muscle that does the same thing on both sides of the body. Well, that's not quite right.

You actually have two hemidiaphragms, one on the left side and one on the right side. These two hemidiaphragms are not the same, as shown in Figure 10-8(a). The right hemidiaphragm is larger than the left and has the advantage of sitting atop the liver, which assists in maintaining the hemidiaphragm's domed shaped. As you've seen, this domed hemidiaphragm position is essential for effective breathing. In contrast, the left hemidiaphragm is smaller and is in an unfavorable, partially-flattened position because the heart is pressing down on top of it,[1] as shown in Figure 10-8(b).

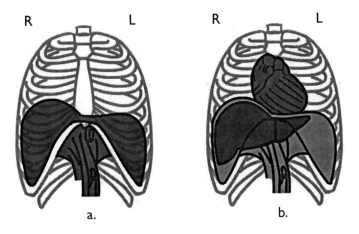

a.   b.

Figure 10-8. (a) The right hemidiaphragm is larger and better positioned for respiration than (b) the left hemidiaphragm, which is smaller and compressed by the heart.

Because of its smaller size and compromised position, the left hemidiaphragm doesn't function as well as the right for respiration. It has a harder time doming back up into a relaxed position, and it tends to stay extended.[1] If you refer back again to Figure 10-2, picture your left side in the extended posture (a) and your right side closer to the optimal posture (b). The right side of the rib cage rotates down and in, while the left side rotates up and out. Thus, the respiratory hemidiaphragm is in a good, domed position on the right, and a poor, extended position on the left. Due to this imbalance, the surrounding muscles become compromised in their position and function, often resulting in a left twist of the rib cage,[10] as shown in Figure 10-9.

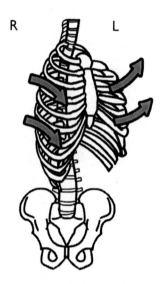

Figure 10-9. The rib cage twists to the left as a consequence of the asymmetrical hemidiaphragms. The right ribs internally rotate, while the left ribs externally rotate.[10]

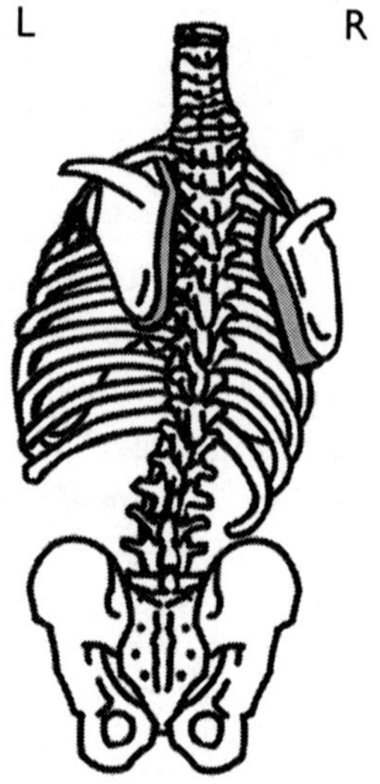

Figure 10-10. The shaded area between the rib cage and scapulae demonstrates the increased gap that is created on the right side when the rib cage twists to the left.

Now here's where it gets really interesting. For efficient breathing, air has to come into each section—front, back, and sides—of the lungs (Figure 10-1). Since the rib cage is internally rotated on the right, it is difficult for the body to inflate this side, especially the top part of the lung. The ribs need to rotate up and out to create the space needed for the lungs to expand. Proper breathing from the hemidiaphragms facilitates this action. However, when the hemidiaphragms are imbalanced and the left is dysfunctional, the body employs another strategy to fill the right chest with air: it uses the accessory muscles—neck, back, shoulder and chest muscles—for respiration. To create more room in the right chest, the neck and shoulder muscles compensate. They lift and rotate the top ribs up and out of the way so that the lungs can expand and air can circulate.[10] I can attest that you will have constant neck and shoulder tension on your right side if you are using this strategy to breathe. At one point, my pain was so bad that I could barely turn my head in either direction. Seeking relief, I had multiple saline injections to calm the muscles, which nearly made me pass out.

This twist in the rib cage not only affects your breathing, but it also impacts shoulder mechanics. You've already heard how breathing changes lower body position. Now I'll describe what happens in the upper body.

The Rib Cage—Shoulder Blade Relationship

My career-ending gymnastics injury in college was chronic right shoulder pain. I'm not talking about just tight muscles like I described earlier. I'm talking about deep joint pain that made it impossible for me to hang from the uneven bars, my favorite event. Despite seeing many professionals, a cause was never determined, aside from some calcium deposits, which seemed unlikely to create my symptoms. It was a mysterious injury that couldn't be solved—until now.

The following is taken from an article by Postural Restoration Institute® (PRI) trained physical therapist Lisa Bartels, DPT, PRC, discussing shoulder injuries in volleyball players:

Once the reader can appreciate the concept of the ribs directing the shoulder blade, and thus directing muscle force couples around the rotator cuff, they will be able to understand why some athletes have a great tendency toward shoulder injury.[11]

To paraphrase, a twisted rib cage affects shoulder blade (scapulae) position, the surrounding muscles, and the integrity of the rotator cuff. When the rib cage twists to the left, the right scapulae loses its underlying support, and the left scapulae position is also altered, as shown in Figure 10-10.

If you've ever been told you have winged shoulder blades, this is a reason why. The left and right shoulder blades are no longer balanced and functioning as designed. According to Bartels, this compromised position and the faulty movement patterns that result set you up for shoulder prob-

body

lems: "Poor suboptimal rib cage and scapular mechanics precedes shoulder dysfunction and pain."[11] Perhaps this asymmetry in my structure was the cause of my right shoulder pain. Performing on the uneven bars requires incredible flexibility and strength in the shoulder. My shoulder was in a poor position, and therefore, was weak and lacking function, making it more susceptible to pain and injury. If I had only known to move my rib cage back into a neutral position, I might have been able to continue to swing happily from the uneven bars. Unfortunately, this was not realized at the time of my injury. Hopefully, it will be addressed for future patients.

Reposition Your Rib Cage

When we address proper upper body position in the thorax region of the body—neck to abdomen—there are two key players: the scapulae and the rib cage. And there are two types of motion regarding the scapulae and rib cage. You can move your scapulae over your rib cage or thorax—Scapular-Thoracic (ST) motion—or you can move your rib cage beneath your scapulae—Thoracic-Scapular (TS) motion. You may be less familiar with TS motion, as I was.

For years, in my own therapy and with my clients and students, I focused on ST motion, diligently moving scapulae atop the thorax by pulling the shoulder blades down and together. I didn't pay much attention to the position of the rib cage below, nor did I consider that it could or even needed to move. But of course it can move. It is held in place by the soft tissues that are adaptable. Unfortunately, sometimes we don't recognize this, since the rib cage seems like a fixed and immobile area of the body.

Therefore, my original approach to repositioning the upper body was incomplete. Although ST motion is needed, TS motion is more crucial. Michael Cantrell, MPT, PRC, Postural Restoration Institute® (PRI) instructor, explains:

Activation of Scapular-Thoracic (ST) musculature without first (or simultaneous) accounting for proper positioning of the Thorax under the Scapulae (TS) is folly since the results would produce neither proper positioning of the scapulae nor the ability to maintain proper positioning of the scapulae if any repositioning occurred.[12]

The scapulae need the support of a well-positioned thorax below to maintain their alignment and function. We need to keep the natural forward rounding in our mid-spine with a well-positioned rib cage to align the upper body.

To untwist the upper body, then, practicing TS exercises is necessary. This movement counters the extended posture described previously—rib cage twisted and flared up and out, more to the left. A variation on the plank exercise shifts the emphasis to TS motion.

Practice Plank Exercises

You can watch a video of this exercise on my website: www.thepfathlete.com/resources.

1. Start on your hands and knees. Your hips should be directly over your knees, and your shoulders should be aligned with your wrists. Feet are hip-width apart, with the toes turned under and relaxed. Exercise is best felt with bare feet. Position your nose so that it is in line with your fingertips.

2. Tuck your pelvis under so that your back rounds up. You should feel your abdominals engage and your lower back lengthen. Hold this contraction for the duration of the exercise.

3. Spread your fingers wide and push your hands firmly into the floor, feeling the primary muscle (serratus anterior) between your rib cage and shoulder blades engage. You are bringing the front of your rib cage down while moving the back of your rib cage up into your shoulder blades, as shown in Figure 10-11(a).

4. Using your respiratory diaphragm and intercostal muscles, breathe in through your nose. As you exhale out through your mouth, press your hands harder into the floor as you reach your rib cage toward the ceiling, and engage your abdominals more. Hold this exhaled position for three seconds before inhaling again. Complete five

body

breaths, then take a brief rest for 10-30 seconds. Perform three to five repetitions.

5. To progress the exercise, extend your legs straight behind you with your toes flexed. Your body will be nearly straight from your ankles to your head while maintaining the rounding in your upper body, as shown in Figure 10-11(b). Start by holding this position for five breaths and three to five repetitions. As you build strength, increase the number of breaths per repetition, up to 20 or more.

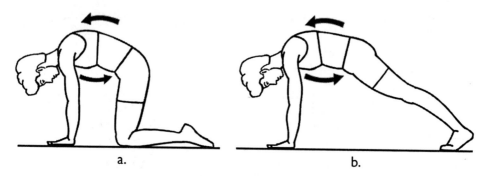

a.   b.

Figure 10-11. When practicing the plank exercise, which emphasizes Thoracic-Scapular (TS) motion, visualize that you are pulling your rib cage down with your abdominals in front and rotating your rib cage up into your scapulae in back.

The Breath and Stress

Repositioning your rib cage improves your ability to breathe efficiently from your respiratory diaphragm, strengthens your core, and reduces your risk for a shoulder injury. What you might not be aware of is this: moving your rib cage to a neutral position can also reduce your stress.

Another consequence of a rotated, twisted and flared rib cage is continuous activation of the sympathetic nervous system (SNS).[10] When the lower part of the rib cage flares up and out in the front, as seen in extended posture, and mainly on the left, the upper portion of the rib cage rotates backward (posteriorly) toward the spine. This sometimes creates the appearance of a hump, most commonly seen on the right side. This rib cage position reduces the posterior space in the thoracic cavity, called the posterior mediastinum, and puts additional pressure on your spinal cord and the sympathetic nerves,[10] as shown in Figure 10-12. Essentially, your twisted upper body posture could be holding you in the SNS.

The SNS invokes the stress response, which prepares you for action—"fight-or-flight." In this state, your body is pumped full of potentially harmful chemicals, mainly epinephrine and cortisol.[13] Symptoms associated with chronic SNS activation include anxiety, fatigue, irritable bowel syndrome, high heart rate, panic-attacks, and more.[13] Repositioning the rib cage, then, takes pressure off these nerves. This allows them to turn off so you can relax and activate the parasympathetic nervous system (PNS). The PNS invokes the relaxation response—reducing blood pressure, heart rate, metabolism and respiration. The relaxation response enhances self-repair with the release of healing chemicals—dopamine, oxytocin and endorphins.[13]

The book *Mind Over Medicine*, by Dr. Lissa Rankin, focuses on the failure to release these healing chemicals when in the SNS. She explains that you cannot heal yourself when you are stuck in the SNS because your self-repair mechanisms are shut down.[14] This reduces your body's ability to repair an injury. It also lowers your capacity to recover from workouts. Thus, turning

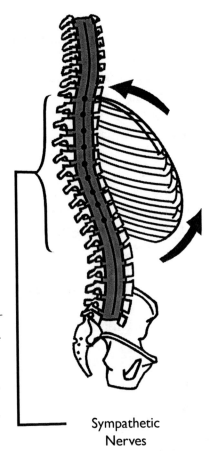

body

Sympathetic Nerves

Figure 10-12. With the rib cage in a rotated, twisted and forward flared position, there is continuous compression on the nerves of the sympathetic nervous system (SNS).[10]

211

on the PNS not only helps you to heal, but it also allows you to train better for your sports.

Physically, it is hard to get out of the SNS, but it may be even more challenging to make the shift in your mind. Our society is full of stressors. The stress response was intended to save our lives when being chased by a large animal or attacked by a vicious tribe. Once the threat passes, the nervous system should return to relaxation.[14] Dogs are good at re-setting their nervous system. After an intense bout of play, you'll often see them shake. This is a stress-relieving action to calm their nervous system.[15] Humans tend to use a deep breath for the same purpose. Unfortunately, we humans are not as good at shaking off the stress as dogs are, and we don't consistently take deep breaths when we need them. Additionally, poor breathing mechanics may be reinforcing activation of the SNS, as just described, thereby counteracting the relaxation we were trying to achieve with our deep breath. We tend to hang on to stress longer than we should. Dr. Rankin tells us that we have *50 or more stress responses a day!* In today's culture, the SNS is activated by threats that are far simpler than losing your life—such as negative thoughts, financial worries, not expressing your creativity, staying in abusive relationships, living in an unsupportive environment, enduring a hated job, lacking life purpose, or feelings of isolation and loneliness.[14] Some of these stressors—negative thoughts, feelings of isolation and loneliness, lacking life purpose—may sound familiar, as they were mentioned in Chapter 3 in association with the stages of grief that many athletes go through when injured.

More proof that healing only happens when we are in the PNS comes from Adriaan Louw, PT, PhD, CSMT, a leading educator in pain science. He points out that the stress response fires your large, strong muscles in order to ready you to fight or flee. Good posture is not a concern in a life-threatening situation. He states that if you are in a prolonged state of stress, you will not respond as well to your therapy.[16] Your body perceives bigger threats to deal with beyond crooked bones and small posture muscles.

My nervous system has definitely settled with regular posture therapy, a surprising benefit of the process. You might recall from Chapter 4 that I fought my wellness coaching mentor when she asked me to take five minutes to sit still and breathe. At that time I refused to comply with her request. I was stuck in the SNS; I couldn't relax, nor did I want to. Now, many years later, I appreciate the benefits of quiet stillness and can sit without moving in relaxation and meditation, being mindful, for much longer than five minutes.

We need to be able to relax in order to heal. In my opinion, many of the modalities we seek for pain relief—massage, acupuncture, meditation, hypnotherapy, yoga and more—attempt to invoke the PNS and our natural ability to heal. In addition to relaxation, we also need to be able to sense our bodies, our environment, and our movements in order to end our chronic pain. Gaining this awareness was the last step in my healing journey, and it is the topic of the next chapter.

body

Summary

Breath is life! The way you breathe directs the position of your core and has postural ramifications for the joints above and below. Breathing with your accessory respiratory muscles—neck, back, shoulder, and chest muscles—compromises the posture of your core by lifting the rib cage up and out from the spine, and extending the lower back into a greater arch as the pelvis tilts too far forward. The misalignment of the pelvis is caused by a combination of tight hip flexors and an extended respiratory diaphragm. The hip flexor muscles—psoas and iliacus—and respiratory diaphragm can be thought of as one long strand of interconnected muscle tissue that works together. This kinetic chain of muscles, the Anterior Interior Chain (AIC), starting with the respiratory diaphragm, extends all the way to the hamstrings. The hamstrings, located in the back of the body, should counter the forward tilting of the pelvis, but will be ineffective if over stretched.

The respiratory diaphragm is divided into two hemidiaphragms on the right and left sides. The right hemidiaphragm is bigger and better positioned for breathing than the left. As a result of this imbalance, the rib cage tends to rotate to the left. Realigning this postural deviation requires moving the rib cage beneath the scapulae in a Thoracic-Scapular (TS) movement, such as the plank exercise.

Many people are stuck in extended posture, which represents a state of inhalation, and they don't fully exhale. A twisted rib cage keeps you locked in a poor position physically and in a stressful state mentally/emotionally. When you are fixed in an extended posture, you are cemented in the Sympathetic Nervous System (SNS). The goal is to attain optimal posture and activate the Parasympathetic Nervous System (PNS). The breath is the key to switching between your nervous systems. The quality of your breath has far-reaching effects on many of your body systems. *Breathe well!*

Game Winning Strategies

1. Learn Correct Breathing Mechanics

You want to learn diaphragmatic breathing, not just for the relaxation benefits, but also for the alignment changes. To watch a video on diaphragm breathing and read about breathing mechanics, visit my website: www.thepfathlete.com. You might also search the Postural Restoration Institute® (PRI) website: www.posturalrestoration.com and consider working with a certified professional in this scientific approach. Providers (like me) and clinics are listed online.

2. Exhale Longer When You Workout

When you're pushing hard during a workout, you might notice that you fall back into a pattern of chest breathing. I do. While exercising, remind yourself to extend your exhale when the intensity increases. I'm not saying to exhale longer than your inhale but to focus on exhaling sufficiently to keep your core muscles strong, aligned and moving. When done correctly, you'll feel a natural rhythm develop. When you're not gasping for air with each breath, your effort should feel easier. Also, you can fool your opponents even when you're suffering, a tip I learned from my husband!

3. Do Rib Cage Repositioning Exercises Often

We are creatures of habit. Your body will revert back to its flared and twisted position if it is not regularly reminded of an alternate posture and efficient function. In this chapter I gave you one example of a rib cage repositioning exercise, the plank, which you can watch on my website. You'll find other examples on my blog. Whatever you choose, do the exercise(s) consistently—before your workouts, after your workouts, as part of your gym routine, and whenever you can.
Plank video: www.thepfathlete.com/resources
Find more rib cage repositioning exercises: www.thepfathlete.com/blog

body

215

11

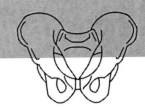

Gaining Sensory Awareness

*T*hrough my physical healing journey, I became aware of my asymmetrical posture, so I practiced exercises to improve my alignment. I gained strength and function in muscles that were dysfunctional; I stopped compensating to move. I realized that I didn't breathe well, so I learned how to use my diaphragm for respiration. As a result of these efforts, I was doing quite well—except for the fact that I still experienced the same nagging back pain I had when I started my therapy. Although my back pain had lessened greatly, it was still there. I was also limited in my sports, and I couldn't cross-country skate ski without pain. Although I was grateful for how far I'd come and what I'd achieved, I believed I could get even better. I wanted it all—complete recovery. I didn't want to settle for giving in to my pain or reducing my activities.

Eventually, my tenacity paid off, and I was successful in my quest. The last piece of my healing involved gaining sensory awareness. This chapter will define what that is as well as the steps I went through to achieve it. As you read this chapter, please note that I will use the terms "sensory awareness," "Somatics," "proprioception," and "kinesthetic awareness" interchangeably, with the same general meaning.

What is Sensory Awareness?

Your senses—taste, touch, sight, smell, and hearing—provide information about your surroundings. They guide you in your interactions with the external world. Being aware of these senses is an inner experience. Thomas Hanna, PhD, who first introduced "Somatics" in the 1980s, refers to this internal knowing of yourself as the soma, which he defines as the "living, self-sensing, internalized perception of oneself."[1] Sensory awareness, or Somatics, is your ability to be aware of the stimuli coming into your body from your environment. This is a very personal process, with the information only being accessible by you, as Dr. Hanna explains: "To yourself, you are a soma. To others you are a body. Only you can perceive yourself as a soma—no one else can do so."[1] This is why I tell my clients that we are partners in their healing. I can observe a client's body, but he is the only one with access to his soma. I cannot experience what a client feels in his body or mind.

The soma refers not only to your physical sensations, but also to your mental and emotional states. For example, through external observation, I cannot feel that your muscle is tight, nor can I know if your mind is confused and anxious. When I was still not completely recovered, no one else could do this analysis for me. I was the only one with access to my soma, and my soma, how I perceived the world through my senses, needed healing.

Sensing Before Movement

If you accidentally put your hand on a hot stove, you'll quickly pull it away to stop the burning. Your body feels an extreme temperature through your sense of touch, and it responds by removing your hand from the danger. Similarly, when the doctor hits your knee with a hammer, your knee involuntarily extends. The hammer stretches your patella tendon, which is sensed by receptors in your tissue, triggering your body to shorten your thigh muscles. Likewise, when lifting a box, you automatically sense its shape and weight so your muscles know how much force to exert. Have you ever picked up an object that was lighter than you expected, only to be thrown off balance as you used too much effort? Your body sensors also tell you how much pressure to use when grasping an object. Squeezing an egg too tightly will spoil breakfast.

These are all examples of how your senses influence your actions. You are constantly reacting to your external surroundings through the information provided by your sensory system: the collective input to the brain from your senses via your nerves. Sensory data allows you to orient and move correctly in space with little effort.[1] Let's imagine that as you're reading this book, you are sitting at a table. On the table, to your right, is a glass of water.

When you reach for the glass of water, your hand easily makes contact. How does this happen? First, you sensed the location of the glass through your peripheral vision (sense of sight). Second, your brain took note of where it was sitting in relation to your body (kinesthetic sense, to be discussed later in this chapter). Third, your brain directed your hand toward the object until it felt the glass (sense of touch). Your correct assessment of the environment as perceived through your senses enabled this successful motion.

Sensory input is especially important for athletes playing sports. When kicking a soccer ball, you need a good sense of the ball's position in space—as well as where your foot should contact the ball and how much force and effort to apply to get the ball in the goal. Football quarterbacks have to gain a broad sense of the field and know where all of the players are before throwing a pass. Running on a technical trail requires extensive feedback from your feet and peripheral vision to navigate without falling. When making a delicate putt, a golfer needs to have a keen sense of how much muscle tension is needed to contact the ball with appropriate pressure to land it in the cup. A gymnast needs a good sense of her orientation to land a flip on a four-inch-wide balance beam.

Sensing comes before movement. Dr. Hanna describes this well in his book, *Somatics*: "We require a constant stream of sensory information from the outside in order to maintain ongoing control of our muscular movements from the inside out."[1] All of the preceding sports movement examples require delicate coordination between your senses and your actions. If your sensory assessment of a situation is "off," you may lose the game, golf match, or gymnastics competition. Sensory miscalculations can also result in injury.

Sensory Input Creates Motor Output

Your brain receives sensory or somatosensory input from specialized peripheral nerves called "sensory receptors." These receptors are located throughout your body in the muscles, tendons, joints, organs, bones, skin, eyes, teeth, inner ear, and more. These receptors monitor pressure, temperature, stretch, force, chemical stimuli, mechanical stress, position, light, vibration, touch, pain, etc.[2] Your receptors relay continuous feedback to the central nervous system (CNS)—brain and spinal cord—through nerve

body

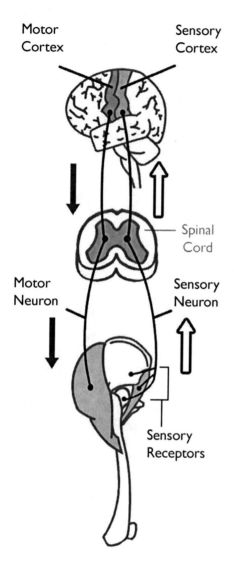

Motor Cortex

Sensory Cortex

Spinal Cord

Motor Neuron

Sensory Neuron

Sensory Receptors

Figure 11-1. Sensory nerves (neurons) bring information to the sensory cortex from the sensory receptors in the body, and motor nerves (neurons) take information from the motor cortex in the brain to the muscles.

impulses to the sensory cortex of the brain, as shown in Figure 11-1. The brain assimilates this information to create awareness of your body's position, speed and direction of movement, and tension throughout your soft tissues. Craig Williamson, MSOT, pioneer of *Somatic Integration*, refers to this as your kinesthetic sense.[3] Your kinesthetic sense is often referred to as your sixth sense.

Adjacent to the sensory cortex of the brain is the motor cortex, which directs movement, as shown in Figure 11-1. These brain areas work in tandem as a feedback loop. In Chapter 8, one-half of this feedback loop was discussed: in Figure 8-8, the motor output side of the loop was portrayed in reference to activation or inhibition of the muscles around the hip. Figure 11-1 completes this loop with the addition of sensory input from the body. Dr. Hanna explains, "The sensory nerves carry to the brain information about what is happening in the world as well as in our bodies. Provided with this information, [...] the brain integrates the incoming sensory information with outgoing commands to the motor system."[1] Physiologically, this is how the senses dictate your movements. Therefore, how well you sense your environment and how well you sense your own body influence your movements and ability to heal.

Traditional Therapy Focuses on Motor Output

Therapists and coaches (myself included) sometimes get it backward, focusing on motor output before sensory input. It is assumed that you have good sensory input, which is often the case—but not always. I followed this typical path in my recovery. Also, as a coach, I assume correct sensory awareness when I ask my clients to contract muscles. When they cannot even feel those muscles, it can be very frustrating and demoralizing for them.

Remember my inability to contract my medial thigh muscle when doing leg lifts? I had no sense of this muscle or how to use it. My brain and body were not in sync. When a muscle is not used for a long time, the neurological connections between the tissues and the brain become weakened. When asked to work, the muscles don't respond because the communication channel with the brain is too faint. Dr. Hanna refers to this as "sensory-motor amnesia."[1]

I often use the term "rewiring" with a client. Together we are literally establishing a new transmission route between the soft tissues and the brain. One of my physical therapists, Torin, used the analogy of paving a dusty dirt road into a superhighway. When injured, the dirt road is the rarely traveled route of correct movement sequencing, while the superhighway is the ingrained behavior of compensated motion. Rewiring lays asphalt on the dirt road to develop the correct high-speed transportation route. Rewiring faulty patterns of movement cannot happen without adequate sensory input. How you perceive this input dictates how you move within the world. Particularly, what you see and feel through your soma affects your posture, movement mechanics, and chronic pain.

Sense-Based Therapy

There are several complementary therapies based on rewiring the soma. I've experienced both the Alexander Technique® and the Feldenkrais Method®. The Alexander Technique® was developed by Frederick Matthias Alexander through self-experiments to cure hoarseness in his voice, a hoarseness so obvious that it threatened to curtail his acting career.[4] By observing himself in the mirror, he noticed that a tension pattern developed every time he spoke. He noticed that the pattern also presented even

body

when he only *thought* about speaking, clearly indicating a mind and body connection. How he thought about speaking, and how he actually spoke, caused tension in his neck, which altered his posture and voice quality.[4] Missy Vineyard, master Alexander Technique® teacher and director of the Alexander Technique School of New England, explains: "Physical sensation was an all-important bridge, linking his body's movements with his mind's perception."[4]

Vineyard refers to this as "flawed proprioception"[4] in her book *How You Stand, How You Move, How You Live.* She explains that the sensory receptors in your body send messages to your brain, which create both mental and physical responses. According to Vineyard, proprioception involves much more than just body awareness. In her view, proprioception also includes knowledge of how you are feeling, from physically moving a body part, to your emotional state, to other sensations such as hunger or being too warm. She states:

> The feelings that are generated within us as we do everything we do—from moving to thinking to remembering—not only shape how we move, they shape our beliefs about ourselves, and this in turn influences our actions and decisions.[4]

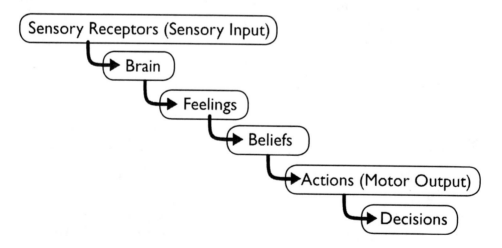

Figure 11-2. A simple depiction of Vineyard's model of proprioception.[4]

The sensory receptors in the body relay information to the brain; the brain then interprets the data and creates feelings. These feelings shape our beliefs, which drive our actions and decisions. Vineyard's description of proprioception expands the feedback loop of sensory input to motor output, as shown in Figure 11-2, to include the intermediary steps of feelings and beliefs.

While in posture class, my student Mary struggled to keep her foot aligned in a straight position. While she was doing an exercise, I corrected her foot position and therefore changed how she sensed her foot through her sensory receptors. Although her foot was now in a straight position, she told me it felt crooked. Altering her foot position caused her to feel her foot differently—and her brain perceived it to be in the wrong position. This incorrect proprioception of her body could elicit many different results. It could influence her to act by moving her foot back to the original lopsided position and continue with the exercise. Or, although it feels incorrect, she could choose to proceed with the exercise in the new foot alignment. Further, because of the inconsistency between how she feels her foot and its position, she might believe that the exercise is not beneficial, causing her to choose to skip it altogether. Finally, she could become discouraged that she isn't doing the exercise correctly, decide that she cannot heal, and stop trying altogether.

body

It is this disconnect between the brain and body, flawed proprioception, that can make it so hard to change a person's position and movement patterns without direct external feedback. Often, what feels correct to us is actually deficient and unbalanced. We typically need external guidance and reassurance so that we can persist in making lasting alignment changes. Remember two of Coral's lessons from Chapter 4: "It's okay to accept help from others," and, "Stay focused on what you want."

The Alexander Technique® (AT) educates you to move with greater mindfulness—awareness of the present moment—and less tension.[5] Working privately with an AT teacher, I learned how to move my body with greater ease: I learned to direct better patterns of muscle engagement while inhibiting (turning off) the unnecessary muscle activation that created tension. Instead of continuously straining to hold myself rigid through my leg, hip, and pelvis muscles—a fear-based protective response—I learned that I could reduce my effort without negative consequences. I could relax my body and mind into a more comfortable position with less stress on my joints. I focused inward on my soma regarding my body tension, and I learned to release my tight restrictions. The result was freer, more fluid movement with less pain.

A couple of years after learning the Alexander Technique®, I had the opportunity to try the Feldenkrais Method®. My first experience was in a class recommended by one of my posture clients.

In a dark room, lying on two mats and a blanket, I was lead through gentle exercises that encouraged me to discover the optimal way of moving. The class exercises broke the movements down to the basics, but they simultaneously demanded unwavering awareness. John, my instructor, would ask things like, where is the movement initiated from within your body? Or, is tension developing in any other part of your body as you move? The exercises were taxing on my brain! The Feldenkrais Method® trains your brain to coordinate with your body better than any online tool could ever do. At one point during class, while lying on my back with my knees bent, I was easily rotating my knees from side to side while rolling my head in the opposing direction. Then John added the instruction to look toward my knees, or in the opposite direction from the rotation of my head. Might sound easy enough, but it wasn't. The next progression required me to rotate my arm inward when my knees dropped to the same side and outward when my knees dropped to the other side. Are you kidding? I'm not this coordinated! This is exactly why I still go to the class every chance I get.

This remarkable class opened my eyes to the profound differences in the way the right and left sides of my body moved. The Feldenkrais Guild's video *What is the Feldenkrais Method?* defines it this way: "The Feldenkrais Method,® [is] an internal journey to rediscover [...] balance, flexibility and coordination."[6]

In class I realized I could not move my left side in the same fluid, unrestricted manner as the right. I felt oh-so-uncoordinated on my left. Before taking the class, I never would have guessed the pain in my hip had such a profound effect on my body communication systems and movement abilities. But it did, and through the class lessons, I learned to integrate my movements much better. With greater body coordination and efficiency, I am faster and more powerful in my sports. This is an objective of the Feldenkrais Method®: "Just as important as building muscle is how all the muscles work together to support the skeleton in action."[6]

Although I found these sense-based therapeutic approaches to be helpful, worthwhile additions to my regimen, they didn't provide the results I was ultimately after. I still had my familiar back pain and skiing limitations. Even though it was beneficial to increase my kinesthetic awareness through my soma, this still was not enough. Sometimes, your senses themselves are flawed and need adjustment. Sometimes, the way you perceive the world is skewed and is delaying your recovery. And sometimes, you need to alter the sensory information coming into your body from your environment. This may mean changes in things like your glasses prescription, foot orthotics, dental splint, or even the input to your ears, which are all areas of research at the Postural Restoration Institute® (PRI).[7] Since vision is the primary sense in the brain, and 80% of the sensory input we receive about posture comes from vision,[8] I'll start the discussion about changing sensory input through this sense.

body

Neurology and Your Eyes

My client Jaqueline was born with a lazy left eye. An accomplished runner, her career was cut short when she suffered a left hamstring/adductor magnus (inner thigh) tendon tear. Years following her injury, she had chronic pain on her right side. She experienced pain in her hip, sacroiliac joint (SIJ), and low back. She also developed plantar fasciitis and shin splints on her right side. Her symptoms migrated up her body, causing tightness in her right neck and serious temporomandibular joint (TMJ) issues. Her biggest source of discomfort, though, had been chronic right psoas (hip flexor) tightness and right groin pain. Despite numerous treatments, she consistently plateaued, stumping her therapists, who could not figure out why she could not get better.

The treatment approach of the Postural Restoration Institute® (PRI) marries sensory input and motor output. PRI practitioners recognize there are higher centers in the body, particularly vision and bite, that can hold patients in painful postures and movement patterns.[7] When Jaqueline and I learned of the Postural Restoration Integrative Multidisciplinary Engaged (PRIME™) program[9] at the Hruska Clinic™, which examines the sensory and motor systems together, we agreed she should go for treatment. This interdisciplinary approach included evaluation by a behavioral optometrist (Dr. Heidi Wise OD, FCOVD), a dentist, a PRI physical therapist (Ron Hruska, MPA, PT) and a Doctor of Podiatric Medicine.[9] Here is Jaqueline's recollection of her visit to the PRI Vision™ Center[10] in Lincoln, Nebraska:

Within the first five minutes they (Ron and Heidi) told me that my problem was "developmental" because of a single entry on my intake form, "born with a lazy left eye." My parents were told that I would grow out of it. However, as Ron and Heidi explained, the body does not grow out of it. Instead it adapts. This is because "lazy eye" is a developmental issue in which the information taken into both eyes is not correctly integrated and processed in the brain. The brain ends up ignoring the input from one eye and preferring the other eye. The eye that is being ignored wanders off in other directions. Eye convergence issues—eyes not working together as a team—can cause problems in coordination, depth perception, and other mobility functions.

Since my left eye was "lazy," my brain ignored its input. The left side of my body was not connecting with my brain. Now this sounds weird since I could walk, and the left side moved perfectly fine. However, the muscles really were not firing but were only moving from muscle memory. When the brain does not sense several crucial muscles that are needed to physically move/walk/run, other muscles incorrectly take over the functioning. Since my right eye became the primary visual source of neurological input to my brain, this created a situation where the right side of my body was constantly in the "on" mode, trying to compensate for the left. The result was that the right side was always tight. This created asymmetry and dysfunction. And pain. The pain from my right psoas tightness was debilitating. It was constant, and it led to all of the issues on my right side that I had experienced. In short, my injuries were all due to my left lazy eye.

Being the skeptical scientist, when I heard this, I was like, "Yeah, riiigght." Ron watched me and pointed out some of the automatic movements that I subconsciously made to allow my left side to communicate with my brain. For example, I constantly touch my hands together. I move from foot to foot, cross my arms, and put my hands in my pockets. To listen, my head tilts to the right and turns to the left, since my right is what is processing (or listening). He was correct. However, although I was intrigued, I was not yet convinced.

Ron and Heidi worked together to generate the best Rx [prescription] for my condition. Ron had me insert a cheap dental splint to keep my teeth from touching asymmetrically while I was being fitted with eyewear. They provided me with a pair of prism glasses that were intended to force my left eye to "turn on" and get my body to realize there is a left side visually, spatially/peripherally, and tactilely. By turning on my left eye and the left side of my body, my overly-worked right side muscles would "turn off." What I experienced was nothing but a sea of change for me—when I put on these glasses and walked, my pain just melted away. The glasses I was given changed my world . . .

body

Jaqueline's sensory input from her visual system was altered with her prism glasses, allowing her to move differently and without pain. She had what Williamson describes as "kinesthetic dysfunction" caused by her vision. In his book, Williamson explains,

If you have kinesthetic dysfunction, you cannot accurately sense whether certain muscles are relaxed or engaged. [...] It is a problem with how you perceive the messages coming from your kinesthetic receptors. You need two things to correct kinesthetic dysfunction: new sensory input and a willingness to pay attention to it.[3]

Like many of us, Jaqueline had spent years trying to change her motor output without regarding or modifying her sensory input. Once her brain received new sensory information through her visual system, her function immediately improved. Since she was perceiving the world differently, her pattern of moving through space changed. As Dr. Wise said in the *Postural Visual Integration* course, "The easiest way to get out of a pattern is to take the pattern away."[8] The glasses took Jaqueline's destructive, painful pattern away.

Vision is More Than Sight

As you read Jaqueline's story, you saw how the prism glasses were designed to help her orient in space and become aware of her left side. There was no mention about how well she could actually see. "Sight" is your ability to see clearly, including your ability to sense your peripheral field. But "sight" is only one component of "vision," even though it is what we associate with "vision" since it's what is typically tested during an eye exam. When you have your eyes checked, it's common that only one visual pathway (out of the eleven that have been documented) is tested. This pathway, from the retina located in the back of the eye to the brain through the optic nerve, concerns itself with how clearly you see. It is included in the central nervous system (CNS). At the PRI Vision™ Center, other visual pathways are tested to determine your integration of proprioceptive information provided through the entire visual system.[8]

On Jaqueline's second trip to the PRI Vision™ Center, I joined her to have myself checked out. I thought my "sight" was pretty good, with only a minor correction for distance. However, upon examination by Dr. Wise and Ron Hruska, I found out that my visual system was flawed in its ability to orient me in space. It was determined that my vision issues were not developmental but behavioral, most likely the result of my many early years as a gymnast. Through my examination it was also determined that when I looked upon the world, I perceived the ground to be sloping away from me. My brain thought I was always going downhill, and my posture adapted accordingly by extending backward so that I didn't tumble down the slope.

Why did I see the world with this optical distortion? It's unclear, but it may be related to stress. In his book *Muscular Retraining for Pain-Free Living,* Williamson refers to an "extension reflex."[3] This reflex is triggered by stress and activation of the sympathetic nervous system (SNS). This involuntary contraction of muscles pulls you backward, away from a perceived threat.[3] So, stress could have been driving my posture and distorting my vision. I am continually amazed at the pervasiveness that stress has on all the body systems.

Regardless of why, the fact remained: I perceived a downhill world. At the PRI Vision™ Center, Ron Hruska affectionately called me a "pixie" because I floated over the ground and could stand on my toes for a long time. I had little sense of the floor, always being light and forward on my feet, rarely on my heels, and bracing for a slide down the hill.

Sense the Ground With Your Heels

Lacking the ability to sense the ground with my heels, I could not move forward without compensation. And it was not enough just to sense the floor—I needed to be able to integrate that sensory information into a healthy pattern of movement. Heel strike is the first phase of the gait (walking) cycle, as shown in Figure 11-3(a), and if you don't get that correct,

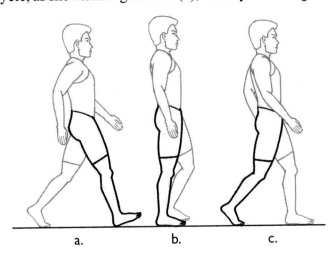

      a.   b.   c.

Figure 11-3. The three phases of the gait cycle, shown on the right leg, are (a) heel strike, (b) mid-stance, and (c) push-off.

everything that follows is going to be wrong. According to Hruska, "the ground is your seventh sense! You can't do anything with kinesthetic sense if you don't know what to do with it in the environment. You have to be able to sense the floor."[8]

Successful heel strike is achieved through your peripheral vision. Awareness of the periphery guides your movements. Peripheral vision helps you to orient yourself in space. Without awareness of my left periphery, I didn't know where I was in relation to my surroundings. Thus, I could not move forward without cheating. *I was literally lost in space!*

Unfortunately, for many of us, our peripheral vision shuts down, particularly on the left side because of our innate asymmetries and right-side dominance, which I will discuss shortly. Our brains are double-wired to notice our surroundings on the right but only have one pathway to process visual information from the left side.[8] To feel my left heel, I had to sense my left peripheral field of vision.

The prism glasses I received at the PRI Vision™ Center helped me to sense my heel on the ground. Specifically, the glasses changed how my brain interpreted my environment. The glasses altered my visual input so that my brain could perceive flat ground as flat, not sloped downward. They also expanded my awareness of my left visual field.

Without the prism glasses, I was missing my seventh sense, the ground. And without the ground, I could not center myself in mid-stance, the second phase of the gait cycle, Figure 11-3(b), nor could I push-off, the third phase of the gait cycle, Figure 11-3(c). Rather, I pulled myself through space with my eyes, hip flexors, and neck. I constantly looked at the ground when I walked. I would fixate on a spot with my eyes, and then I would move myself forward through over-activation of the muscles on the front side of my body—hip flexors and neck. Ideally, I would be pushing myself through space by activating muscles on the back side of my body, specifically my hamstrings and gluteal muscles. We want to push, not pull, ourselves to move forward.[8]

Our vision can provide postural stability. Each of our eyeballs is surrounded by six skeletal muscles call the extraocular eye muscles (EOMs). The primary job of the EOMs is to move the eyeball in its socket. However, these muscles are 300 times stronger than they need to be to move the eyeball.[8] This extra strength can be used for stability. Since I couldn't feel the ground when I walked, I looked at it intently to orient and steady myself in space. Staring at the ground and using the EOMs to stabilize the body is the number one vision problem seen at the PRI Vision™ Center. For many people, vision is the primary sense holding them up.[8] This is why it can be so much harder to balance with your eyes closed.

Sensing the floor through your heels requires activation of the muscles on the back side of the body—hamstrings and gluteals.[8] Now back to my point about overstretched hamstrings. When tested, my hamstrings easily went far past 90 to around 110 degrees (Figure 11-4). This excessive flexibility was impacting my ability to find the ground and contract my hamstrings. It was my number one issue. Creating awareness and strength in these muscles became the main emphasis of my PRI therapy program.

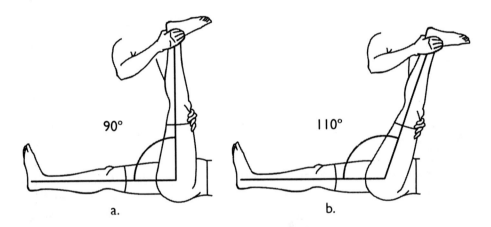

Figure 11-4. (a) Healthy hamstring flexibility is 90 degrees. (b) My hamstrings had excessive flexibility, stretching to 110 degrees.

At the PRI Vision™ Center, it took some drastic measures for me to sense my left heel and hamstrings. In addition to wearing training glasses to correct my optical distortion, weight was strapped around my midsection to increase my mass; a special brace (Protonics X1)[7] designed to engage my hamstrings was put around my left leg; and I was given more supportive footwear and orthotics. Picture that for a moment! Fortunately, using all these devices, I finally received the sensory input I needed to sense the ground. Whew! And, once this was accomplished, my hamstring length returned to the desired 90-degrees. These devices created new sensory input and

body

movement patterns, which activated and shortened my hamstrings while walking.

My therapeutic exercises, done while wearing my prism glasses, were based on creating strength and awareness in my left leg—heel, hamstrings, inner thigh, and glutes—in coordination with my left abdominals. I had to be able to balance on one foot at a time, as required during the mid-stance of gait, with appropriate muscle activation. And, I had to be able to do this on both sides of my body alternately as I stepped one foot in front of the other. Believe me, it sounds easier than it is when you can't sense correctly or use your muscles appropriately.

With this new perception of the world, provided through my PRI Vision™ prism glasses, I could finally stop extending backward to steady myself. This reduced my pain and changed my dysfunctional movement patterns. Now that I had proper muscle engagement, I could find my left heel. Hurrah!

Lost Proprioception Causes Injuries

Remember back in Chapter 5 when I warned about taping and bracing body parts? Well, here's why. It was my left ankle that had been taped for many of my gymnastics years. By continuously bracing this part of my body, I had lost sense of my foot. Now with the tape off, I didn't have a clue where it was in space or how to stand on it correctly. You know what it feels like when you try to walk on your foot when it's asleep? Imagine having that lack of sensory input all the time. Your body will have to cheat to move.

If you have ever had an ankle sprain, you may have gone to physical therapy—and there, you may have used a wobble board. The purpose of this balance exercise is not just to strengthen the stabilizing soft tissues, but also to enhance proprioception. During my time as a physical therapy assistant, one thing I learned is that you lose your ability to sense the position of your foot in space with an ankle sprain injury. This lack of awareness makes it more likely you'll step down on the foot incorrectly again and suffer another sprain, which frequently happens. A recurrent ankle injury is not necessarily a strength issue. It is often one of proprioception. It is important to point out that this same principle also applies to injuries in other parts of your body.

Right Side Dominance

As humans, we tend to be dominant on the right side. It is not by chance that most of us are right-handed; this is a pattern. Ron Hruska, MPA, PT and founder of the Postural Restoration Institute® (PRI), has expanded the science that links internal asymmetries in the human body, right-sided dominance patterns, and postural changes that lead to pain and disability.[7] Internally, we have more organ mass on the right side of our body. For starters, we have a larger right hemidiaphragm, which was discussed in Chapter 10. Additionally, our liver is also on our right side. Recall how the liver sits under the right hemidiaphragm and assists in keeping it in a functionally domed position. We also have an extra lobe of lung on our right side. Finally, our brain is lateralized, with specific functions residing on the right and left hemispheres.[11]

The left hemisphere of our brain specializes in speech and language, while the right hemisphere specializes in processing nonverbal information and spatial relationships.[12] For simplicity, you can think of the left hemisphere as logical and the right hemisphere as creative. In the late 1800s, the French physician Pierre Paul Broca discovered brain localization while working with patients who had limited speech abilities. Autopsies of these patients showed lesions in the left hemispheres of their brains. This area of the brain is now referred to as Broca's area, and speech loss due to a legion in this area is known as Broca's aphasia.[12]

The left brain hemisphere controls our muscles and movements on the right, and the right brain hemisphere controls the left.[13] Therefore, handedness—if you are dominant with your right or left hand—is a function of brain lateralization.[13] In addition, the brain itself is asymmetrical, with the right hemisphere protruding forward, while the left hemisphere is positioned rearward.[13,14] Most people, 90-95% of us, are dominant in our left brain hemisphere for language and are right handed.[13] This dominance of the left brain hemisphere predisposes us to a pattern of using the right side of our body, including preferring our right hand and standing on our right leg.[11] Consider the environment we have created. It is tailored for right-handed people—doorknobs are on the right, tools are designed for use with the right hand, car stick shifts (at least in the U.S.) are on the right, etc. Approximately 70% of left-handed people are also left-brain dominant for language.[13] And,

body

they share the same internal asymmetries in their structure as right-handed people, making them prone to the same dysfunctional patterns.

Wondering if you are biased to your right side? Observing your daily movements can reveal your tendencies. For instance, do you find yourself standing and shifting your weight to your right leg more than your left? When sitting, do you tend to cross your left leg over your right, rotating your pelvis to the right (right-side bias), or right over left, rotating your pelvis left (left-side bias)? While sleeping, do you find yourself rotating your pelvis right or left? For example, when you sleep on your left side, is your left knee ahead of (right-side bias) or behind (left-side bias) your right knee?

Transferring your weight to your right leg is a normal, healthy pattern. The problem is when you are stuck on the right side, like I was, and are unable to go to the left side correctly. When this happens, the left lower body musculature becomes weaker and less functional than the right from disuse. When I was addressing my right-side bias tendencies noted in the prior questions, the hardest one for me to change was the last one: I really struggled to get comfortable with my pelvis rotated left to sleep. Many of us cannot shift back into our left hip like we can our right hip.[11] My body had to learn to use my left hip and build strength in the supporting musculature.

Balancing the Body Through Counter Rotation

Remember in Chapter 10 when I told you the rib cage twisted to the left due to the asymmetries in our hemidiaphragms? Well, often, in order to counterbalance, the lower body twists to the right, as shown in Figure 11-5. This is what the body naturally does when we walk and are in mid-stance on our right leg: the right hip rotates back, the pelvis turns to the right, and the upper body counter-rotates to the left.[11]

Before I go any further, it should be noted that this pattern that I have described—with the pelvis twisted right and rib cage twisted left—is a typical pattern seen in clients with pain and injury, but it is not exclusive. There are more patterns that can be layered on top, causing a person's posture to look different from what I have stated. Each person is unique and should be treated as such. However, the fundamental pattern I have described tends to underlie additional dysfunctions and compensations.[8] And, as I mentioned, this counter-rotated pattern is a normal and healthy part of the gait cycle. The problem occurs when we cannot reciprocate—we cannot do the same on the left leg: the left hip rotates back, the pelvis turns to the left, and the upper body counter-rotates to the right. When I watch people walk, run, and even cycle, I often see good lower body rotation to the right and upper body rotation to the left, but I notice that the pelvis and upper body only make it back to the center and never rotate in the opposing directions—pelvis to the left and upper body to the right.

Besides not being able to move evenly when walking, a person can become stuck in this twisted posture all the time. I have seen this in myself and in a number of my clients. When I am stationary, my body is in this twisted position, with my pelvis turned to the right and my upper body counter-rotated to the left. To release this pattern and to move symmetrically from side to side with gait, the appropriate muscles need to turn *on* and *off*. Many of my muscles perpetually had the *on* switch flipped and never powered down. These muscles included those in the Left Anterior Interior Chain (Left AIC), introduced in Chapter 10. The Left AIC muscles—left hemidiaphragm, left hip flexors, left tensor fasciae latae (TFL), left lateral quadricep and left hamstring—are swing chain muscles, which means they should be turned *on*

R   L

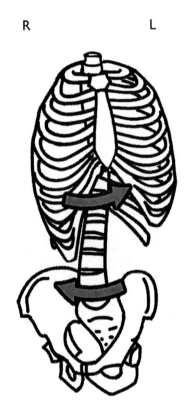

Figure 11-5. A left twist of the rib cage often accompanies a right twist of the pelvis.

body

235

when the left foot is off the ground during the gait cycle, as shown in Figure 11-6(a), and turned *off* when the left foot is on the ground.[8]

In my body, however, with overactive Left AIC muscles, these left swing chain muscles remained *on* when I was standing on my left leg, as shown in Figure 11-6(b). When standing on my left leg, my left stance muscles should be active. If I could not inhibit or turn *off* these left swing chain muscles, I would be perpetually biased to my right side and my right leg, with my pelvis turned to the right, even when my left leg was in contact with the ground and my pelvis should be turned left. When my left swing chain muscles were *on,* I couldn't rotate and shift my hip back into left stance. This is why the pelvis often does not rotate back to the left. It only makes it to the centerline of the body, as described previously.

Since my left side swing chain muscles (Left AIC) did not turn *off,* my right side stance muscles were also always engaged. The right-side stance muscles include the muscles surrounding the hip and low back. *And where was my never-ending back pain and skiing hip tightness?* On my right side, the side I was always standing on, even when my left foot was on the floor. To end my back tightness and ski without pain, I needed to be able to turn *off* my right side stance muscles

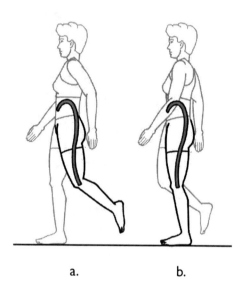

a.   b.

Figure 11-6. (a) The left swing chain muscles (Left AIC), highlighted in the image, should only be *on* when the left leg is off the ground. (b) The Left AIC remains *on* in left mid-stance, which is a dysfunctional pattern.[8]

and turn *on* my right swing chain muscles. Simultaneously, I needed to be able to turn *off* my left swing chain muscles (Left AIC) and turn *on* my left stance muscles. And here's where the hamstrings come into the picture—again. Hamstrings, particularly the more medial muscles (there are three hamstrings), are left stance muscles. To be able to achieve the stance phase of gait on my left leg, I needed to be able to feel my left hamstrings. And, to feel my left hamstrings, I needed to sense the ground with my left heel.[8]

Sensing a New Reference

The Postural Restoration Institute® (PRI) refers to certain parts of the body as "reference centers." You can also think of these areas of the body as "contact points" or "stabilization centers." Three of these reference centers are the left heel, the right medial arch, and the left ischial tuberosity (sit bone).[15] If you cannot feel these reference centers, you will not be able to sequence your muscles correctly for movement. You will lack the ability to turn *on* the appropriate muscles and turn *off* the opposing muscles. Developing new references is essential for creating a lasting change in position and motion. Otherwise, the body reverts back to its previous reference centers, unbalanced position, and faulty biomechanics.[15]

If I could not feel my left heel and activate my left hamstrings while simultaneously letting go of my right lower back reference, I wasn't going to overcome the pain in my right lower back, nor was I going to move efficiently. In an illogical way, I wanted to feel pain in my low back. It was helping me to stabilize my body. It was where I sensed contact. Recall from Chapter 8 that the body gains stability through impingement. My impingement site was my right lower back. To recover, I needed a new impingement site. And, according to Hruska, that site should be my heel on the ground. As he states, "The hardest impingement you need in life is the ground."[15] To help me sense and impinge on the ground with my left heel, I was fitted with custom PRI orthotics for my shoes. These orthotics were not to stabilize my feet, but rather to help me create correct kinesthetic awareness. The feet need to wobble to function, not to be locked in place. The heel bone, or calcaneus, has the largest sensory area of any bone, making it neurologically highly connected with the brain. My foot orthotics were guiding me to an optimal foot position so I could sense and impinge the ground.[15] Body

body

stability should come from sensing the heel contact with the ground, not pain in your back.

The right medial arch is also a reference center. Sensing the right medial arch brings the foot into a more neutral position (Figure 11-7[b]), and it helps rotate the body to the left so you can sense and impinge on the left heel. Awareness of the right medial arch can be gained through contact of the right heel and right big toe. When I would skate ski, I had a habit of rotating my right foot onto the outside lateral edge, known as supination, and lifting my big toe (Figure 11-7[c]). In this foot position, I was not able to move off my right side and shift over to my left side, which overtaxed my right hip muscles and made them tighter and tighter as I skied. Supination on the right foot lifts the right medial arch, which is an important reference center for correct body mechanics. To skate ski without pain, I had to develop proprioception of my right medial arch.

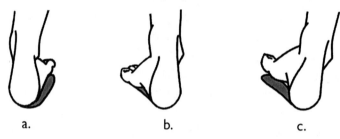

a.   b.   c.

Figure 11-7. The right foot is shown in (a) pronated, (b) neutral, and (c) supinated foot positions.

Through my therapy, I became aware of my tendency to hang out on the outside edge of my right foot. *Pronation,* rolling the foot inward so that you can sense your medial arch, *is not bad!* This is shown in Figure 11-7(a). Actually, it is needed for correct impingement at the ankle, as I explained in Chapter 8. For review, remember that stability in the feet, which translates into stability in the joints above, is created when the medial foot bones contact each other. Stable feet improve neuromuscular patterns and reduce pain.[15]

I had been told that I overpronate, so I purposely avoided allowing my feet to rotate inward. Consequently, I forced myself into a position of supination, and, as a result, had no awareness of my big toes. This kept my body in an unstable position. I didn't have the stability coming up from the ground and feet as I should, so I found support by impinging in other places: namely, my right lower back.

Neurology and Your Teeth

Vision helps your proprioception. It guides you to find the right position and reference centers. As my physical therapist Torin at the Hruska Clinic™ further explained, this new-found posture is held or lost contingent on your bite, which stimulates the sensory receptors in your mouth. When you biomechanically bring your teeth together, a process called "occlusion," the sensors in your mouth that respond to pressure are activated. The process has widespread effects throughout your body systems.[16] This is why Jaqueline mentioned using a dental splint to keep her bite aligned and teeth touching evenly on the left and the right sides during her PRI Vision™ treatment. If she had been allowed to go back into her original bite, her posture would have negatively changed. Let me explain.

I have worn a lot of dental devices throughout my life—retainers, spacers, braces, rubber bands, neck gear, and headgear. Basically, if the dentist or orthodontist thought they could fit something into my mouth, they did. Could all this tinkering in my mouth have been connected to my pain? Well, yes! What often happens in the quest to straighten the teeth is that the bite is altered. When the teeth don't line up and come together evenly, posture can be affected. Just hearing about all the orthodontia I had made Raulan, my PRI physical therapist, sweat. My bite triggered an unhealthy pattern in my body, which Raulan discovered while conducting joint mobility tests: when he initially tried to move my right shoulder, he found that it had limited internal rotation. My left hip was also fixed in position, lacking the ability to adduct (move inward toward the body). Additionally, my neck had limited rotation to the left. We tried various exercises to gain mobility, and Raulan even did some manual releases—hands-on stretching and repositioning techniques. There was some improvement but nothing remarkable. Lacking progress, he suspected there might be something higher in the nervous system driving my position—my bite. What? He had me bite down and

body

asked me where the molars contacted first: on the right side, as he suspected. Like my pelvis, my jaw was also rotated to the right. Then he stuck a tongue depressor in my mouth and instructed me to bite down on my left side and take a few breaths. Okay? That's all he did—no exercises, no manual releases, just breathing. We retested: my right shoulder swung forward with ease, my left hip adducted, allowing my knee to drop to the table, and my neck had full range of motion without pain. REALLY? I was in shock. I couldn't believe the changes. How was this possible?

My bite pattern was setting off a negative sequence of events in my body that affected the tension in my muscles and joints. When my teeth came together (sensory input), the resultant pressure sensed in the receptors of my mouth sent a message to my brain. The brain, then, relayed this information to my spinal nerves, which changed the length and tension in my muscles (motor output), altering my posture.[16] As I learned in the PRI *Cervical Revolution* course, "feedback from proprioceptive nerves in [the area surrounding] teeth and the temporomandibular joints (TMJ) govern the creation of neural pathways, which in turn determine the <u>duration</u> and <u>force</u> of overall muscle activation needed for postural stability and performance."[14] Every time my teeth touched in my old pattern, with the right side contacting first, the tone of many of my muscles increased, and my joints—right shoulder, left hip, and cervical spine of my neck—became locked in their previously-learned and restricted positions.

Also of importance in my experience are these facts: I am a jaw clencher and tooth grinder at night; I have been diagnosed with Temporomandibular Disorder (TMD); and I have tension on the right side of my neck. The right side of my jaw pops often and occasionally locks up, making it hard for me to open my mouth and chew food. This is written in the present tense since I am still working to correct these issues. Several years before seeing Raulan, I had been supplied with a mouth guard to protect my teeth from the grinding. As I discussed in the last chapter, some of my right neck tension was attributable to my breathing pattern, but there is more to the story. The sensory receptors in the neck muscles are highly sensitive to the head's position and movement.[14] My head is forward and twisted.

While at the PRI Vision™ Center, I had to stare at my face in a mirror and notice how asymmetrical it was. That was fun—NOT! I don't recommend it. Like with the rib cage, we incorrectly assume that the bones in the head are fixed. However, with a twisted skull, my cervical muscles are unbalanced, and my neck position is compromised. A couple of years earlier, a chiropractor told me my neck was "military straight," meaning it lacked natural curvature. The point of all this is that my neck and jaw problems are largely stemming from my uneven bite and lack of contact on my left teeth.

Working with Raulan, I was fitted with a new dental splint. This would not only protect my teeth from clenching and grinding like my previous one did, but more importantly, it would reset my bite with balanced occlusion on the left and right sides. Aligning my teeth to contact evenly on both sides of my mouth provided my brain with a new reference. Changing this input kept my body from reverting back to its old pattern and allowed my shoulder, hip, and neck to stay in a neutral position. I continue to work on this by wearing my dental splint at night, observing and correcting my clenching tendencies during the day (which I fix by putting my tongue on the top of my mouth), and practicing daily alignment exercises to further improve my position and function. Maybe someday I will be free of my dental splint—or I'll at least stop breaking them! (I've had eight and counting.) The good news is that they are lasting longer as my pattern improves.

body

Higher neurological centers, such as the eyes and jaw, dictate how muscles behave. The Postural Restoration Institute® (PRI) maintains that when therapy is unsuccessful, it is likely that sensory issues with vision or occlusion are blocking progress.[14]

Sensory Awareness Aids Healing

After learning about my tendency to overuse my right side and to walk on the outside edge of that foot, I was able to use this intelligence to my benefit during a duathlon race. This is what happened when I started hiking uphill after a long hill climb on my mountain bike:

I hurt from the first step. I had no pain during the bike ride, but suddenly, my right hip was screaming. What was I going to do? Stop and turn around, or push on? Tuning into my body mechanics, I paid attention to how my right foot was contacting the ground and how that affected my hip pain. Soon, I found that I was landing on the outside of my right foot, which sent instant pain into my right hip. If, however, I focused on stepping on my whole foot, putting weight on the inside edge, feeling my right heel, big toe, and arch while engaging my inner leg muscles, my pain subsided. Taking deliberate balanced steps, my pain continued to lessen, and I finished the race.

Once I was able to sense my left side and had the strength and coordination to use it equally with the right, most of my remaining symptoms went away. The last piece of my healing journey required a neurological shift. After years of motor output-based therapy, I was astonished at how quickly I improved when I altered my sensory input and acquired new references. We are designed to alternate smoothly from right to left, but many of us get stuck on our right side for different reasons. Not only does our ability to reciprocate easily from side to side benefit our bodies, it also enhances our minds.

Recall that our brains are divided into right and left hemispheres. If we are physically anchored in the right side of our body, we are also rooted in the left side of our brain.[14] The left side of the brain is the logical and analytical side. I would agree that this is where my mind tends to be focused. Alternatively, the right side of the brain thrives on being creative and artistic. Definitely not my strength. By learning to physically go into the left side of my body, I opened up communication with the right side of my brain, which assisted me in my writing. As I said at the beginning of the book, our body systems are interrelated at every level.[7]

Summary

Successful rehabilitation and injury prevention should incorporate sensory input along with motor output. Traditional approaches to healing are heavily focused on motor output. The information coming into the body through your senses impacts how you perceive your environment and move within it. You are the only one with access to the sensory information within your soma, which includes both awareness of your physical body and knowledge of your mental and emotional states.

Complementary therapies such as the Alexander Technique® and the Feldenkrais Method® emphasize sensing before movement. However, sometimes your senses are flawed, so your perception of the world needs to be changed with modifications, such as eyewear.

To move correctly and without pain, you must first be able to orient in space. This comes from your proprioception, primarily vision and touch—contact with the ground and between your teeth. Of primary importance is having awareness of your left peripheral vision, which is often lost due to the right-side dominance pattern of the human body. Brain lateralization and internal asymmetries in the body bias most people to the right side.

Second, you need to impinge—make intentional contact—with the ground by sensing appropriate references when you walk. Specifically, you need to sense your left heel and right medial arch. If you do not gain body stability by sensing these correct reference centers, alternative impingement sites will be found, such as the lower back. How you see the world and how you sense (feel) your reference points impact the function and sequencing of your muscles.

When walking, a smooth transition (heel strike, mid-stance, push-off) occurs by appropriately turning muscles *on* and *off* alternately between the right and left sides. However, many people are stuck in a twisted posture, unable to inhibit the swing chain muscles on the left (Left AIC) that keep the pelvis turned right and upper body turned left. They lack the ability to counter-rotate in the opposite direction—pelvis turned left and upper body turned right. The ability to reciprocate between the right and left sides is essential for the health of your body and mind.

body

Game Winning Strategies

1. **Enhance Your Sensory Awareness**

   Become more connected with your body and what you are sensing. You can join a class, hire a private instructor, or just carefully observe your movements.

2. **Sense Heel Contact**

   Correct gait movement starts with heel strike. Make sure you are hitting your heel first and not landing on your toes when you walk. Following heel strike, roll through mid-stance and sense that you push-off over all five toes. In particular, feel your big toe in contact with the ground as your heel lifts prior to stepping forward.

3. **Keep Your Head Up**

   As you move throughout your day, keep your eyes on the horizon, not on the floor in front of you. You can see more than you think with your peripheral vision. You don't always need to look down to see objects in your path.

4. **Train Your Left Peripheral Vision**

   When you are walking, pay attention to what is on your left side. You will not see these objects clearly. Rather, you just need to have awareness of them. As you are moving forward, whether walking, running, Nordic skiing, or hiking, observe yourself passing objects on your left. Pick an object to your left side in the distance and notice yourself moving in front of it.

5. <u>Swing Your Arms</u>

As you take a step forward, your pelvis and upper body should counter rotate. With your right foot forward, your pelvis should turn toward your back (left) leg while your upper body turns right, in the opposite direction. Arm swing facilitates this counter rotation though the body. When the right foot is forward, the left arm is forward, encouraging the upper body to twist to this side. When you walk, notice that both of your arms are swinging equally in front of and behind your body, encouraging this natural rotation.

6. <u>Commit to a Treatment Path</u>

Now that you've heard my entire story, it is time for you to start on your healing journey. *What do you choose for your treatment path?* If you are torn between a few, make a pros and cons list for each. Once you have made your selection, consider the first step you need to take. Then, set a timeline for this action.

body

3

Align Your Training

12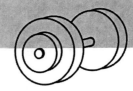

Developing Functional Strength

To play sports and avoid injury and pain, you must be strong. What does that mean, to have a strong body? We often define strength as the ability to lift heavy weights or to apply great force. The problem with this definition is that it does not account for HOW a body accomplishes these feats. Squatting 600 pounds is only impressive if it is done with good form, can be repeated, and doesn't cause pain or injury. The Egoscue Method® defines functional strength as the "ability to retain structural integrity with little to no compensatory motions necessary under duress."[1] It is evaluated by the following three criteria, and it includes the absence of pain: (1) Perform a task properly, free of compensatory motions. (2) Repeat the movement successively with little degradation in performance. (3) Remain injury-free via the proper mechanics and use of the body according to its design.[1]

Functional strength and movement come from a stable and aligned posture. When you are in a good position, your muscles can produce the most power, your joints have full range of motion, and you move with ease and grace. With a balanced structure, you will easily meet the previously-listed criteria for a functional strength evaluation. Unfortunately, athletes of all levels tend to lack function and alignment. You can be dysfunctionally strong and participate in sports at a high level, but this will be short-lived, as it was for me. The body cannot endure compensation and dysfunction in combination with the extreme demands of sports for long, as Pete Egoscue points out:

> Elite athletes can be dysfunctional. Talent, skill and ability in a specific sport by a specific individual can overcome and make up for many dysfunctions. In fact, many of the sports gifted athletes are incredibly dysfunctional. Their bodies have developed sports

specific compensations. Unfortunately, physical performance does not tolerate dysfunction. That is why, over time, so many athletes lose their skills and/or end up playing in pain.[1]

To enjoy an extended, pain-free athletic career, you must be functionally strong.

What is Functional Strength?

Functional strength means being strong in the movements and positions used in sports. To gain these abilities, the body must be trained the way it is used in sports. As you will read, functional training incorporates many of the concepts I've already discussed in reference to aligning and healing your body. Vern Gambetta, internationally recognized expert on sports training and conditioning, and Gary Gray, PT, FAFS, developer of Applied Functional Science® and founder of the Gray Institute®, explain the essence of function:

> Function involves the body's osseous [bone] system that provides structure [posture], the muscular system that provides control, and the proprioceptive system [body and sensory awareness] that coordinates and directs movement, all of which are profoundly affected by gravity, ground reaction forces, and momentum. Where functional stability is concerned, isolated strength gains are minimized and the neuromuscular system [wiring efficient body mechanics] is emphasized.[2]

Functional training, then, takes what you have learned and gained through rehabilitation, and it increases the intensity to make it more applicable to sports. It is not sports-specific training, however. Michael Boyle, strength and conditioning pioneer and top expert in sports performance training, actually calls it "sports-general" training.[3] There is a misconception that functional training means doing movements that mimic your sport. In actuality, functional training focuses on the five basic human movements: (1) rotational and spiral, (2) pulling, (3) pushing, (4) single-leg, and (5) bend-and-lift.[3] These movements are consistent across sports.

As an example, let's consider the basic human movement of single-leg strength and balance. Can you think of an athlete who performs with her feet on the ground who doesn't need this ability? From soccer goalies kicking a ball, to ice skaters landing a jump, to any sport requiring running, being able to stand strong and balanced on one leg is essential. Even golfers and baseball pitchers need to transfer their weight from the back to the front foot and balance on their finishing leg.

Because of these commonalities across sports, similar functional training movements can be used by each athlete. The workout is tailored to an individual sport by placing emphasis on the movements most relevant to the athlete's sport. For example, rotational and spiral movements aren't of high concern to a bobsled pilot who focuses more of his efforts on pushing exercises. The workouts of divers, tennis players, and ballet dancers, however, place a sizable emphasis on rotational and spiral movements.

This chapter gives you an introduction to the concepts of functional strength training with guidance on how to get started. As with the rest of this book, I'm not going to give you a specific plan, but I will provide information for you to consider in developing your strength training program.

Get Straight, Then Strengthen

"Get Straight, Then Strengthen"[1] is a phrase I learned during my Egoscue® training. The meaning is clear. You first need to be aligned before adding resistance to your body. You don't want to strengthen a crooked position and dysfunctional or compensated muscle biomechanics.

This applies to strength training as well as athletics, in general. Lifting weights and playing sports are both strengthening exercises for your body. A set of bench presses and a mile run both ingrain movement patterns and build strength in the muscles used. It is important to make sure you are developing functional, not dysfunctional, power. If done in an unbalanced position, these activities further accelerate the atrophy of your postural muscles and skeletal misalignments—not to mention the negative impact poor weight-training form has on your sports performance, as I experienced with my cross-country skiing.

training

I was very diligent about my strength training routine. Twice a week I performed squats, step-ups, and lunges, all the lifts I thought would help my sports performance. The fact that I couldn't keep my knee facing straight forward instead of collapsing inward while executing these exercises was puzzling, but I did the best I could and pushed ahead. I now realize that my movements were grossly compensated, but at the time I didn't know any better, and I didn't care. Scary, considering my occupation as a fitness professional. I was getting stronger, which was my goal. Besides, I could still do everything I wanted pretty well, or so I thought . . .

I learned differently during a fall cross-country ski camp. I knew I had never had great balance on my cross-country skate skis, especially on my right side, and I was jealous of my husband Ken's smooth and seemingly effortless technique. However, I thought I was doing fine—until I watched a video of myself skate skiing. I was appalled by what I saw. Our small circle of advanced skiers and instructors stared at the video screen, perplexed. What was I doing? Skiing, I guess, but it just didn't look right—where my knees should go out, they went in, and my upper body was twisting around to counterbalance . . . It looked awful. Picture an egg beater with its blades rapidly rotating inward and outward. That will give you the idea of what my legs looked like. Ugly! Although I could ski, it definitely wasn't well or graceful. Improperly working with the weights while using poor form had unfortunately strengthened my compensations.

Your body is always trying to help you and to facilitate your ability to do what you want. I wanted to ski, so my body figured out a movement sequence and fired muscles to make that happen. The result was compensated patterns of motion, decreased performance, and escalating pain. To heal and develop functional strength, I had to stop heavy weight lifting and start retraining my muscles with simple movements like I discussed in Chapter 8. I also had to change my mindset about how to gain the function and power I desired. As a Certified Strength and Conditioning Specialist (CSCS), I had it in my mind that I had to push heavy resistance to improve. I thought that was the only route to strength gains. However, as I mentioned in Chapter 11, it is not just the size of your muscles that matters, but the coordination and neurological control you have over your muscles and movements that impacts sports performance. These abilities are most efficient when built on an aligned structure.

Alignment is the Foundation of Strength and Athletics

Gray Cook, MSPT, OCS, CSCS, researcher, national lecturer, and author, developed the "Optimum Performance Pyramid" as a model to understand movement. It is a three-tier pyramid; the large base level is labeled "functional movement," which is topped by "functional performance," and at the apex, "functional skill."[4]

I like Cook's model. I agree that all athletes, regardless of sport, should be able to perform functional movements at the base of the pyramid before engaging in more complex activities. However, I am inclined to modify his pyramid and add a bottom layer for physical alignment, which would include proper joint position and muscle biomechanics, as shown in my "Sports Training Pyramid" (Figure 12-1).

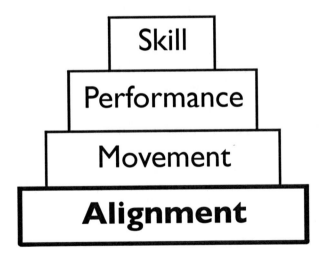

Figure 12-1. The Sports Training Pyramid has alignment as the foundation.

training

Cook explains the base of his pyramid, Functional Movement: "The first level represents the foundation: mobility and stability, or the ability to move through fundamental patterns."[4] In my opinion, mobility and stability, as well as executing proper movement patterns, cannot be successfully attained if the body is out of position and lacks the capability to isolate muscles correctly before coordinating them into patterns, as I discussed in Chapter 8. This is why I've added Alignment to the base of my Sports Training Pyramid.

Remember, it is the *position and condition* of the body brought into sport that matters. Physical alignment is the infrastructure upon which all other work should be built—weight lifting, aerobic exercise, intervals, plyometrics, etc. The second and third levels of Cook's pyramid are focused on performance: moving efficiently with power and specific sports skills. To attain success in these higher levels, the athlete's foundation—physical alignment—must be strong. Otherwise, training plateaus and injury may be inevitable.

A client once asked me why, when training for long distance trail running races, his body would consistently begin to fail around 20 miles into his workouts. He just couldn't pass the 20-mile mark without injury. I explained how he was missing the structural base and biomechanics needed to support longer efforts. He lacked physical alignment; he did not have the proper position and essential muscle engagement patterns necessary to sustain the prolonged running performance he desired. His body could cheat for a while, up to 20 miles, but after that it began to decline. His compensations could only take him so far until his body made him stop. Pain and injury are the body's way of making us take notice.

Stability Training

Prior to adding resistance to your body, you need to be in good alignment. Each day before I exercise, regardless of the activity, I perform restorative movements that enhance my body's alignment and function. These techniques reposition my joints and turn on muscles that tend to shut down, like my left gluteal muscles. These exercises are individually tailored for my body. Although I'd like to skip this pre-exercise routine on some days, I generally don't, knowing the positive impact it has on my performance and injury risk.

Even though muscle activation exercises, like the ones I do and those described in Chapter 8, are routinely used for rehabilitation, some coaches believe they should also be included in an athlete's conditioning program as part of the warm-up. Michael Boyle believes, and I concur, that there are three areas in need of frequent stability training: (1) the abdominal muscles (transverse abdominis and internal obliques), (2) stabilizing muscles of the shoulder blades, and (3) hip rotators (think glutes) and abductors (outer hip muscles that move the leg away from the body).[3] Although the hip joint is generally dominant in mobility, the surrounding muscles need stability to hold the hip in a good position within the pelvic girdle. Alignment in the hip impacts nearby joints, as Boyle points out: "function at the ankle, knee and hip is maximized when the hip displays greater stability."[3]

So that you can take this advice, what follows are some stability exercises addressing these three areas. While you are already familiar with two of the exercises since they were described in previous chapters, I have made modifications here to incorporate the hip musculature. The final exercise is done in the more functional standing position, preparing you for standing exercises and enhancing your proprioception. I'd recommend starting with these before your strength training workout in the order presented. These exercises are adapted from the Egoscue Method® and Postural Restoration Institute® (PRI).

Stability Exercises

Three stability exercises are provided: (1) pelvic tilt exercise with strap, (2) plank exercise with strap, and (3) standing knee press and shoulder blade contraction. Videos of all of these exercises can be viewed on my website: www.thepfathlete.com/resources.

In Chapters 9 and 10, I introduced two movements that are both excellent stabilization exercises for the abdominals: pelvic tilts, as shown in Figure 9-15, and the hands and knees/plank, as shown in Figure 10-11. The hands and knees/plank exercise also stabilizes the shoulder blades. The hip

training

musculature can be added to both exercises by including a non-elastic strap placed above the knees. A belt, tied dog leash, or yoga strap all work well for these exercises.

Pelvic Tilt Exercise With Strap

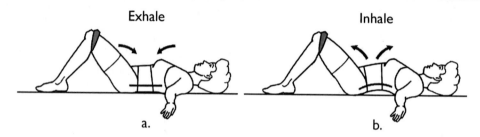

Exhale   Inhale

a.   b.

Figure 12-2. Adding the strap to the pelvic tilt exercise engages the hip rotators and abductors.

1. Place a non-elastic strap just above your knees, as shown in Figure 12-2.

2. Lie on the ground with your knees bent at 90 degrees and your upper body relaxed, arms out to your sides with your palms up. Adjust the strap so your knees are slightly inside your hips. When you push out evenly with your knees, your hips and knees should be vertically aligned. You don't want your knees going outside your hips.

3. Press out on the strap to engage your hip abductor and rotator muscles. You should feel the muscles engaging on the sides and backs of your hips. Hold a moderate pressure on the strap for the duration of the exercise.

4. Maintain sensory awareness of your heels and big toes without pushing into the ground for proper alignment of the feet, knees, and hips. There is a tendency for the feet to roll out, which is why you need to keep the big toes down. This is best felt with bare feet.

5. Start the movement by tilting your pelvis gently up toward your head so that your lower back lengthens and flattens into the ground while your rib cage rotates down in front (anterior). Your lower anterior ribs will come closer to the front of your pelvis. Simultaneously, your posterior rib cage rotates up and backward, so that your upper back ribs move closer to your scapulae and press harder into the floor just below your shoulder blades, as shown in Figure 12-3. Watch that your shoulders do not round forward. As you tilt your pelvis, push your knees forward slightly to engage your deep transverse abdominis (TA) muscle. Avoid over-contracting your rectus abdominis ("six-pack muscle"). Keep this muscle relaxed.

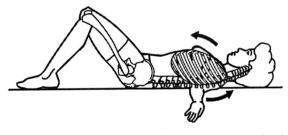

Figure 12-3. The rib cage rotates to flatten the lower back.

6. Next, tilt your pelvis forward toward your heels. Your lower back will lift off the ground into an arch, as shown in Figure 12-2(b).

   NOTE: The movement of the pelvis during this exercise is accomplished by using the surrounding muscles—abdominals, back and hips—and not by simply lifting and lowering your lumbar spine. Strive to feel the different muscles engage as you tilt your pelvis back and forth.

7. Coordinate the movement with your breathing: exhale out through your mouth as you flatten your back (Figure 12-2[a]), and inhale through your nose as you arch your back (Figure 12-2[b]). You'll feel your TA and oblique abdominals engage to pull your ribs down, back and in as you exhale and flatten your back to the floor. One

training

of the under-appreciated but essential roles of your abdominals is forced exhalation. *Your abdominals are exhalation muscles.*

NOTE: Inhaling through your nose with your lips touching and tongue on the top of your mouth facilitates correct head, jaw and neck posture without over activating the neck muscles. Exhaling out your mouth during the exercise enhances contraction of the core muscles.

8. Integrate the pelvic diaphragm muscles into this exercise by pulling up gently with these muscles (similar to what you would do as though you were stopping the flow of urine) as you exhale. Become aware of the natural movement of your pelvic diaphragm in response to your breath on inhale—moving down and lengthening—and exhale—lifting and shortening.

9. Hold the exhaled/back flat position for three seconds with your abdominals engaged before moving into the arch.

10. Repeat this exercise 10-30 times.

Plank Exercise With Strap

1. Place a non-elastic strap just above your knees.

2. Start on your hands and knees. Your hips should be directly over your knees, and your shoulders should be aligned with your wrists. Adjust the strap so that your hips and knees are aligned when you press outward. Feet are hip-width apart, with the toes turned under and relaxed. Exercise is best felt with bare feet. Position your nose so that it is in line with your fingertips.

3. Tuck your pelvis under so that your back rounds up. You should feel your abdominals engage and your lower back lengthen. Hold this contraction for the duration of the exercise.

4. Press out on the strap to engage your hip abductor and rotator muscles. Hold a moderate pressure on the strap for the duration of the exercise.

5. Spread your fingers wide and push your hands firmly into the floor, feeling the primary muscle (serratus anterior) between your rib cage and shoulder blades engage. You are bringing the front of your rib cage down while moving the back of your rib cage up into your shoulder blades, as shown in Figure 12-4(a).

6. Using your respiratory diaphragm and intercostal muscles, breathe in through your nose. As you exhale out through your mouth, press your hands harder into the floor as you reach your rib cage toward the ceiling, and engage your abdominals more. Hold this exhaled position for three seconds before inhaling again. Complete five breaths, then take a brief rest for 10-30 seconds. Perform three to five repetitions.

7. To progress the exercise, extend your legs straight behind you with your toes flexed. Your body will be nearly straight from your ankles to your head while maintaining the rounding in your upper body, as shown in Figure 12-4(b). Start by holding this position for five breaths and three to five repetitions. As you build strength, increase the number of breaths per repetition, up to 20 or more.

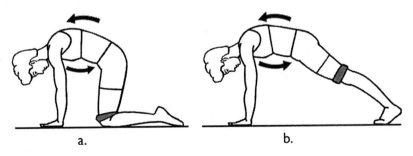

a.   b.

training

Figure 12-4. Adding the strap to the plank exercise engages the hip rotators and abductors.

Standing Knee Press and Shoulder Blade Contraction

1. Place a non-elastic strap just above your knees and stand with your back to the wall. Position your feet so they are hip-width apart and are pointing straight ahead. The strap should be adjusted so that when you press out on the strap, your hips, knees, and ankles are vertically aligned. When standing against the wall, your heels, butt and upper back should be in contact with the wall. If you feel as though you are going to fall forward, move your heels out slightly. Your head may or may not be on the wall, depending on your upper body posture. Keep your chin level to the ground as shown in Figure 12-5(a), don't strain your neck to make your head touch the wall.

2. While maintaining sensory awareness of your heels and big toes, best felt in bare feet, press your knees out against the strap to engage your hip rotator and abductor muscles. You should feel tension and muscle engagement on the outside and back of your hips. Hold a moderate pressure on the strap for the duration of the exercise.

3. Align your core—rib cage over pelvis—by taking a deep breath from your diaphragm. Upon exhale gently engage your abdominals (TA and obliques) by pulling the front of your rib cage down, back and in. You should feel the back of your rib cage, a few inches below your shoulder blades, in contact with the wall. Maintain this alignment throughout the exercise.

4. Gently push your shoulder blades down toward the floor, as shown in Figure 12-5(b). You may feel a stretching in the front of your chest and shoulders and near your neck as you do this. Next, squeeze your shoulder blades in toward your spine, as shown in Figure 12-5(c). You should feel tension develop between the shoulder blades, *not* up toward your neck. If you feel your neck tense, drop your head forward, chin toward your chest. If you still feel your neck tense, just focus on pushing your shoulder blades down to start. Also, be sure to initiate the movement with the muscles in your back, not by moving your arms backward. Keep your thumbs facing forward and your arms relaxed at your sides.

5. Complete 10 slow repetitions, holding each contraction for three seconds.

6. Perform the exercise in sequence with your breathing. Exhale as you bring the shoulder blades together and inhale as you relax and recover. Pay close attention to your core alignment as you pinch your shoulder blades together. Many people will unknowingly raise their chest and extend their lower back when pinching their shoulder blades, thus losing their core alignment. Exhaling on the contraction helps to keep you in a good vertical posture. Complete one to three sets of 10 repetitions.

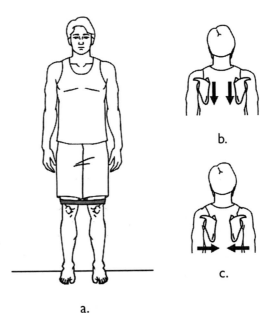

Figure 12-5. This exercise targets all of the recommended stabilizing muscles—transverse abdominis (TA) and internal obliques, shoulder blade stabilizers, and hip rotators and abductors.

The shoulder blade contraction you just learned is something you can mix into your day anytime—driving to work, washing dishes, waiting in line. The more you practice, the easier it becomes. You'll also want to incorporate this shoulder blade movement into your weightlifting workout. Before any lift—upper or lower body—you'll want to pinch your shoulder blades together lightly to set them into a stable position. This will improve your alignment and reduce your chance of a shoulder injury.

training

Strengthen From the Inside Out

"Work from the Inside Out"[5] is another phrase I picked up during my Egoscue® posture training. As I mentioned in Chapter 9, strengthening begins at your core. When talking about being strong from the inside out, a balanced and aligned core is the imperative first step. Beginning your workout with the previous stability exercises gives you a good start, with proper core alignment and muscle engagement.

These core and stability muscles lie deep within your body, closest to the bones and encircling the joints. According to Rolf Wirhed, Fil Lic, author, coach and leading Swedish professor in Anatomy and Biomechanics, these posture muscles are the most critical for injury prevention. He states, "Of all the muscles that protect the joint from injury, those that directly surround it are the most important. A strong and supple musculature is always the best protection against joint injuries."[6]

Muscle atrophy and dysfunction happens from the inside out. Consequently, the positional muscles that are at the most inner layer become weak and ineffective first. When your infrastructure becomes compromised, the supporting rebar that should be providing your stability is failing. Like the grains of sand that create a delicate castle on the beach, your bones are left unsupported. They move too much and into unfavorable positions, leaving you more prone to chronic pain and injury.

Interestingly, traditional resistance training strengthens the body from the outside in. Standard weight lifting exercises target the large, superficial muscles (chest, back, shoulders)—the muscles you can see in the mirror and easily touch. Strength is developed in these surface tissues, while the deeper layers are neglected. External strength can only stabilize your joints so much if the underlying tissues are weak. Essentially, you are creating a hard exterior with a softer, weaker interior. This arrangement makes sense for a walnut that needs a hard shell to protect the tender food inside, but not for the human body. We need to be strong throughout.

The fitness industry has realized this gap and has embraced the idea of core strengthening, as discussed in Chapter 9. Yoga and Pilates have also blossomed in response to this "inner-strength-building" movement. Many of us view yoga as a recovery tool, if you will, something that we should do and that will be good for us. This idea comes from the sports world through our coaches, magazine articles, fellow athletes, sportscasters, and various other sources—blogs, podcasts, etc. We have the perception that yoga and Pilates are gentle and easy, requiring little effort. Although some styles of yoga would fit this description and are very relaxing, many yoga and Pilates classes are demanding, more than most athletes realize. You need to be in good position with adequate function to safely maneuver into many of the required poses. So, although both forms of exercise are generally beneficial, they might not be appropriate for everyone.

A physical therapist friend, Mike, encouraged me to do yoga in my pursuit of healing. This seemed like a great suggestion, so I eagerly attended classes. After giving it my best for several months, I had to stop. I left my last yoga class in tears. It was more than my body could handle. It was making my pain worse. Now I realize that all the hamstring stretches and back extension exercises in the yoga class were contradictory to what my body needed, thus exaggerating my postural asymmetries, muscle imbalances, dysfunctions and compensations. Before I could successfully do yoga, I needed to get straight and improve my biomechanics.

I am not alone; I now see many yoga dropouts in my office. Personalized posture therapy teaches these clients posture and movement basics, which oftentimes are not covered in group classes. Learning these fundamentals helps these motivated athletes get back to their yoga and Pilates classes or daily practice, if desired.

Apply Load to Concentric and Eccentric Contractions

Recall in Chapter 5, Figure 5-1, where I discussed the traditional view of muscles working as a system of levers and pulleys. The idea is that muscles attach to two points, generally two bones, and work in opposing pairs. When muscles are stimulated by a nerve, they shorten, while the opposing muscles lengthen to produce movement. The example in Chapter 5 used the muscles in the upper arm—biceps and triceps—located on different sides of the body. When doing a biceps curl, the biceps muscles on the front of

training

the arm shorten, or contract, and the triceps muscles on the back of the arm lengthen, or are inhibited, when the arm moves upward.

Using this model as the basis for strength building has led to the creation of traditional weight training machines that isolate single-joint movements, such as triceps extensions, leg curls, calf raises, etc. These machines are generally used exclusively to load muscles when shortening, during the concentric contraction, and they provide no resistance when lengthening during the eccentric contraction. On a calf raise, for example, there is only resistance when you push up against the weight as your calves shorten and strengthen. Eccentric loading of the muscles can be done if the weight is lowered slowly against the resistance. Unfortunately, this is not what I observe at the gym, where the weight stack is usually rapidly dropped after each lift.

Weight machines are excellent for rehabilitation, to isolate specific muscles so that strength can be regained. Machines might also be appropriate for the targeted muscle development that bodybuilders need. Also, the technology of these machines continues to improve. However, these segregated motions do not reflect how the body functions during nearly all sports movements. You now know the body works as an integrated whole when it moves. So, why wouldn't you strengthen your body using this concept? *You absolutely would!*

Additionally, this simplified view and bias toward muscle shortening neglects to consider the action performed by muscles when they are lengthening. We think of the hamstrings shortening to bend the knee in a concentric contraction. But what happens when the hamstrings tighten in a lengthened position during an eccentric contraction? What is their function in a long position? Do the muscles have an equally important role during a lengthened contraction, a role that often isn't considered?

For the answers to these questions, I'll refer again to Gary Gray. In the 1990s, Gray introduced a new way of thinking about muscles and movement. He referred to the interrelated actions of the muscles throughout the body as a "chain reaction."[7] Gray applied the concept of kinetic chains, introduced in Chapter 5, to sports movements. Michael Boyle, in his book *Functional Training for Sports*, summarizes Gray's idea of the "chain reaction" response that happens when landing a running stride:

When the foot hits the ground, every muscle from the trunk down has one simple function. The muscles of the lower body (glutes, quads, hamstrings) all act together to stop the ankle, knee and hip from bending in order to prevent falling to the ground.[3]

In this case, the hamstrings are lengthening to prevent the knee and hip from bending. This eccentric contraction of the hamstrings is critical to efficient running mechanics.

Muscles do have an equally important role when contracting in a lengthened position! Strengthening eccentric movements is one of the essential components of functional training. Tri-planar conditioning, discussed next, is another.

Tri-planar Conditioning: Moving in Three Planes of Motion

Another misconception about muscle function is that it occurs in only one plane of movement. Actually, human movement happens in three planes of motion—*Sagittal, Frontal,* and *Transverse* (Figure 12-6).

Most often, we move in the sagittal plane, which splits the body into right and left halves. Imagine a vertical line being drawn down your body between your eyes, splitting your torso and separating your left leg and arm on one side from the right leg and arm on the other. We think of the body flexing forward and extending backward in this plane of motion. Nodding your head in agreement is a sagittal plane

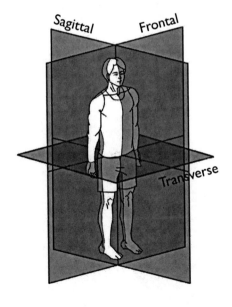

Figure 12-6. We move in three planes of motion.

training

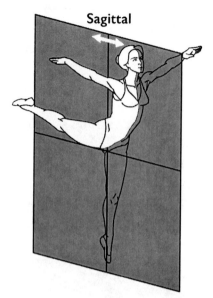

Figure 12-7. When performing a scale, the dancer's body moves in the *Sagittal* plane.

Figure 12-8. When performing a side kick, the martial artist's body moves in the *Frontal* plane.

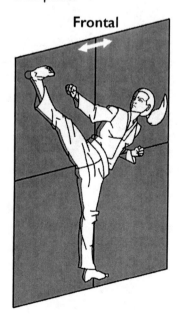

motion. A dancer's scale, where the leg goes back and the upper body goes forward, is also a sagittal plane movement (Figure 12-7).

The frontal plane divides the body sideways into front and back halves. This imaginary vertical line runs down the sides of your body, separating your chest muscles from your back muscles, and splitting your legs and arms into front and back portions. Side-to-side maneuvers (abduction and adduction) take place in this plane of motion. Shifting weight sideways and bending your head side to side are common frontal plane motions. A side kick in martial arts is also a frontal plane movement (Figure 12-8).

The transverse plane divides the body into upper and lower halves. Imagine a horizontal line drawn through your midsection, separating your pelvis, legs, and feet from your torso, arms, and head. Rotation occurs in the transverse plane. Rotating your head to look left and right, or a golf or tennis swing, is a transverse plane movement (Figure 12-9).

Hopefully, you are questioning my sports movement examples right now. I did when I was first introduced to these concepts. The question to consider is—do these actions actually only happen in one

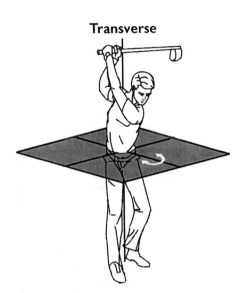

Transverse

Figure 12-9. When performing a golf swing, the golfer's body moves in the *Transverse* plane.

plane? What is the movement of your hip during a golf swing? Doesn't it flex in the sagittal plane, move sideways in the frontal plane, and also rotate? *Human movement is a tri-planar activity!*[7] Now, I need to revise my previous statement. Human movement happens in three planes of motion—*Sagittal, Frontal* and *Transverse*—AT THE SAME TIME. Hence, you need to develop strength in all three planes of motion simultaneously. This is best done by training movements.

Train Movements, Not Individual Muscles

Sports performance is the result of coordinated movements. Casting a fly rod, spiking a volleyball, paddling a boat, skiing moguls, and hiking up a mountain all require multiple muscles working together in a specific sequence to create action. As a general rule, muscles and joints do not work separately and, therefore, should not be trained in isolation. Rather, they work in a "chain reaction," as Gray described earlier, using the body as a unit. According to Vern Gambetta and Gary Gray, "Training individual muscles isolates and breaks the kinetic chain. Training movements integrates and improves the function of the kinetic chain."[2]

Let's take an example of strength training for your quadriceps, the muscles on the front of your thighs. One option to build quadriceps strength is the quadriceps extension exercise, where you are seated in a machine lifting a weight (Figure 12-10).

This exercise isolates the quadriceps by extending the knee joint. There is little to no involvement from the hip above, ankle below, or opposing hamstrings muscles on the back of the leg. But think about this: in sports

training

267

and life, there are not going to be many instances where you are only using your quadriceps muscles to straighten your knee while seated with your feet off the ground. And worse yet, in many endurance sports, you are not going to be using your quadriceps together in the same motion. Rather, one leg will be going forward while the other is going back, as seen in snowshoeing (Figure 12-11).

A more functional free weight exercise for developing quadriceps strength is a lunge on the ground (Figure 12-12). Unlike the quadriceps extension machine, the lunge incorporates many joints and muscles that work together simultaneously to produce a fluid movement. The lunge is weight bearing, another key aspect of functional training discussed next, and requires proprioception, balance, postural alignment, tri-planar movement, and eccentric contractions. Many variations and additional challenges can be added to the lunge exercise as your strength, balance, and coordination improve. For example, you could place an unstable surface like a Bosu ball under your front or back foot. Upper body rotation and resistance could also be incorporated. In fact, there are numerous possibilities. I chose this example to demonstrate the fundamental differences

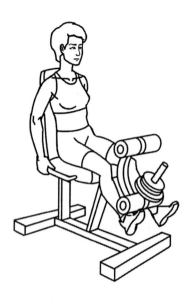

Figure 12-10. The quadriceps extension machine is a single-joint, non-weight bearing exercise.

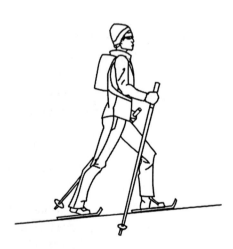

Figure 12-11. When snowshoeing up a hill, the quadriceps are being used in a split-stance position, with one leg forward and one leg back.

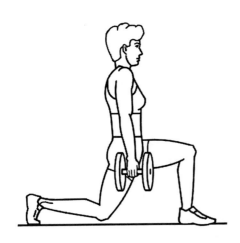

between standard strength training and functional strength training, an isolated muscle approach versus an integrated movement approach.

Figure 12-12. The lunge closely mimics the demands of life and sports.

Keep Your Feet on the Ground

In the debate of machines versus free weights, you already know my opinion: I recommend free weights because they are more functional. Free weights are versatile, require stabilizing muscles to fire, demand bilateral work from the body, incorporate balance, enhance proprioception, and can more easily simulate athletic and everyday movements, which are all important components of functional training.

Free weight exercises also connect you with the ground in many cases, which is essential when simulating tri-planar sports movements for the lower body. Boyle states it this way: "To exercise a muscle as it will be used, you need to close the chain and allow the muscles to work as they would when the foot is on the ground."[3] Many strength training machines have the legs hanging free in the air, like on the quadriceps extension machine in Figure 12-10.

The floor also provides sensory awareness and impingement, as discussed in Chapter 11. In connection with the optical system, the ground gives you a reference and helps you orient in space. Remember how I depicted the floor as your seventh sense in Chapter 11, following kinesthesia, your sixth sense? When standing and moving unsupported on the floor, as you do in most sports activities, you are also responding to gravity and ground reaction forces, adjusting your posture into correct core alignment (Chapter 9), while responding to vertical loads (Chapter 6).

training

Exhale as You Lift

Recall the words of Julie Wiebe, BSc, MPT in Chapter 9, "blow before you go." She gives this advice to activate the core musculature—respiratory diaphragm, pelvic diaphragm, and transverse abdominis (TA)—and to stabilize your center before movement. I would like to modify her statement to—blow *AS* you go. Exhaling out through your mouth as you move against resistance helps to ensure good core alignment and strength through abdominal and pelvic diaphragm muscle engagement. The goal is to be in a neutral posture, with the rib cage coming down in front and the lower back lengthening, especially when building strength. You might want to review Figure 10-2 depicting extended and optimal posture. Exhaling as you move helps to ensure good core alignment through muscle engagement.

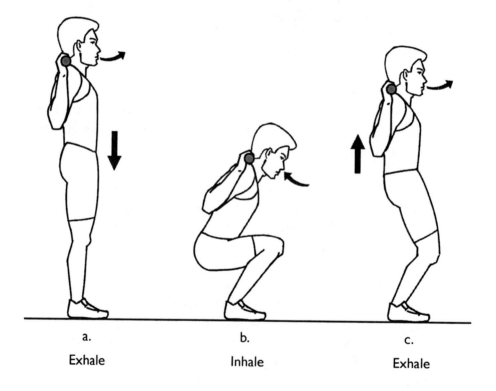

a.   b.   c.

Exhale   Inhale   Exhale

Figure 12-13. Proper squatting technique includes exhaling when lowering and lifting the weight.

Let's take the example of a free weight squat, another functional exercise to build quadriceps strength, as shown in Figure 12-13. Standing with a weighted bar on your back, dumbbells in your hands, or just against your own body weight, you want to exhale as you squat down and lower yourself toward the ground, as shown in Figure 12-13(a). If you consider the quadriceps muscles, this is the eccentric (lengthening) phase of the exercise. At the bottom of the lift, inhale, as shown in Figure 12-13(b), and as you push back up to standing during the concentric (shortening) phase of the lift for the quadriceps, exhale again,[8] as shown in Figure 12-13(c). Alternatively, if you do not want to pause at the bottom of the lift to inhale, start with a small exhale on the way down, followed by a more powerful exhale as you stand back up.[9] This modification still maintains the principle of exhalation on exertion.

Let's consider for a moment that many people claim to hurt their backs when bending over. What are the back muscles doing when you bend forward? They are working in a lengthened position while performing an eccentric contraction. Unfortunately, many of us have overdeveloped our backs with concentric contractions that shorten these muscles as a result of performing exercises like squatting with an overly arched back, lifted chest, and held breath. This leaves our trunk muscles imbalanced and prone to injury. The integration of proper breathing mechanics with lifting facilitates correct alignment and symmetrical muscular development.

Putting it All Together: Patch Fitness®

Patch Fitness® is the functional training program based on the Egoscue Method®.[10] It started as an obstacle course in a tomato patch. (Hence the name.) The concept behind Patch Fitness® is getting you to play like you did when you were a kid, by returning to the fundamental movements the body was designed to do—crawl, duck, leap, climb, jump, etc. A Patch workout incorporates forward, backward, and sideways movements. You go over, under, and around obstacles and push your limits, all while having a great time.[10]

A Patch workout starts with alignment exercises to improve position and increase mobility and stability before strengthening. These workouts follow the principles discussed earlier by Gary Gray, Vern Gambetta, and

training

271

Michael Boyle. Patch workouts include all the components of functional strength—aligned posture, eccentric contractions, moving against gravity and ground reaction forces in a standing position, tri-planar and multi-joint movements, keeping your feet on the ground (most of the time), proprioception, and unstable environments. These workouts challenge the body, just like athletics do.

Professional National Football League athlete John Lynch, former all-pro safety for the Denver Broncos, had this to say about Patch Fitness®: "I believe a large part of my success in the NFL is directly related to Pete Egoscue, the Egoscue Method® and Patch Fitness®."[11] Another distinguished football player Troy Polamalu, former Strong Safety for the Pittsburgh Steelers, also followed a functional fitness program. I only know about Polamalu because of my husband, who is a big Pittsburgh Steelers fan. He loves to sing to me during the season, "Are you ready for some football?" He laughs while I smirk and count the months until it's over.

Polamalu's atypical offseason strengthening program took him back to the Sports Lab in Orange County, CA, to train with the unconventional conditioning approach of his coach Marv Marinovich. In the Pittsburgh Post-Gazette article, "Steelers OK Polamalu's Alternative Training Plans,"[12] Ed Bouchette writes, "Marinovich preaches to athletes to forget all the typical weight-training advice they've received in high school, college and the pros, because it often contributes to injuries and does not prepare them for the speed of their game."[12] According to Marinovich, "When you train slow, it makes you slow. The thing I try to do now is train the nervous system and produce greater force faster."[12]

To get ready for the football season, Polamalu would use wobble boards, stability balls, weighted shoes and light weights of twenty pounds or less as his tools for functional training. He focused on range of motion, stretching, and quick, explosive power. Although his program was radical by NFL standards, it worked for him, from his college days at the University of Southern California (USC) through his NFL career. In 2010, he received the NFL Defensive Player of the Year Award from the Associated Press after a close XLV Super Bowl loss to the Green Bay Packers.

A Patch Fitness® workout is a functional workout! And, although this type of resistance training may not be mainstream in professional sports yet, Lynch and Polamalu have shown that it works at the highest levels in the NFL. Elite athletes in basketball, baseball, golf, volleyball and tennis have also benefited from Patch Fitness.®[11] If it works for these athletes, I expect *it will work for you, too!* It did for me, although I was hesitant to try it myself, fearing pain and injury. Here's my recollection of my Patch Fitness® instructor training class in San Diego.

As I sat at the table looking at two very fit guys, I was anxious. This was a "hands-on" class. I would have to do exercises that I wasn't sure I was ready for. What if I felt pain and couldn't do it? I had to challenge my fears and limitations—big time. We started inside, jumping over static objects that were progressively moved farther and farther out in front of me. My breathing became shallow, my heart raced, and I worried I would hurt myself. However, I jumped the obstacles and received incredible encouragement and support from not only my instructor, but also my classmates. Next, we moved outside, where my body continued to be pushed. As time went on, I felt better, stronger, and pain free. I reflexively kicked into a hand-stand like I used to when I was young but had been hesitant to try. When we finished, we were all exhilarated! What fun to act and feel like a kid again!

My reluctance to physically push myself was mainly in my mind. My body was stronger than I believed. Patch Fitness® encourages you to confront your fears and bust through your self-imposed boundaries to remove limitations.[11] Now, my strength program, and what I recommend to my clients, is functionally based. I love the freedom these workouts offer, allowing any environment to be a setting for conditioning—the beach, a local park, or your backyard. You can be creative in what you do. The only requirement is to use your natural patterns of movement. This is our design; this is how we should move and grow stronger, not by using isolating muscle machines. Start with small changes in your routine and build on them gradually. Functional training is more demanding than typical strength training in many ways, so be patient with yourself. The rewards and enjoyment are worth it.

Strength is only one aspect of sports training. The next chapter introduces the other elements in a wholistic model, one that focuses on training the whole athlete in all the areas that are important for excellence in sport.

training

Summary

Functional strength means being strong in the movements and positions used in sports. Alignment is the foundation of functional strength and the Sports Training Pyramid. Functional training focuses on the fundamental human movements, which translates to all sports. Stabilization exercises for alignment and muscle activation are recommended for the abdominals, shoulder blades and hips as part of your warm-up. These movements will improve your position and function, preparing you for higher demand activities.

Functional strength starts with an aligned core. You need to be strong from the inside out and to move from a well-aligned, solid, and stable center. Otherwise, your body will compensate, and you will be prone to injury and chronic pain. Exhaling while you lift encourages correct core alignment and provides internal stability. Improper lifting technique can carry over into sports technique with dire consequences.

Functional strength is achieved through functional training, combining:

Posture—get straight, then strengthen

Proprioception—incorporate body and sensory awareness

Eccentric (lengthening) Loads—strengthen muscles in a long position

Multi-Joint and Tri-Planar Movements—"chain reaction" of the body

Standing Exercises—contact and impinge the floor with your feet

Gravity and Ground Reaction Forces—created with upright movement

External Instability (unstable surfaces)—to develop internal stability

Patch Fitness® combines these elements into a fun and challenging workout. By simulating the demands of sport, functional training prepares the body for repetitive athletic movements while reducing the chance of injury and elevating performance.

Game Winning Strategies

1. <u>Align Your Body Before Adding Resistance</u>

Prior to your workout, practice stability exercises for the abdominals, shoulder blades, and hip rotators and abductors. Three exercises were provided in this chapter—(1) pelvic tilt exercise with strap, (2) plank exercise with strap, and (3) standing knee press and shoulder blade contraction. Videos of all of these exercises can be viewed on my website: www.thepfathlete.com/resources.

2. <u>Try Patch Fitness</u>®

Visit www.egoscue.com/patchfitness//Videos.htm to watch videos and download exercise handouts. You'll get a great workout and are guaranteed to smile and laugh.

3. <u>Attend a Functional Strength Training Class</u>

Inquire at your local health club, fitness center, YMCA, etc. about functional strength training class offerings.

4. <u>Develop a Personalized Functional Fitness Program</u>

I encourage you to find a certified trainer to develop a personalized program. Consider someone trained by Egoscue University®, the Gray Institute®, or the Postural Restoration Institute®.

I offer all these services at The Pain Free Athlete: www.thepfathlete.com.

training

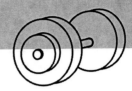

13

Wholistic Sports Training

*T*raditional sports training focuses nearly exclusively on the physical demands of the game. Baseball, football, soccer, basketball, and squash players hit and throw balls for hours. Ice skaters, dancers, gymnasts, divers, and synchronized swimmers rehearse the same moves over and over until their execution is perfect every time. Runners, cyclists, Nordic skiers, rowers, and triathletes spend most of their training hours doing a sport for long durations.

Pick up most any self-training book for an endurance sport and you'll most likely find three-quarters of the pages devoted to physical training and workouts—long slow distance, intervals, sprints, lactate threshold, VO_2max, anaerobic endurance, force, power—the list goes on. A few books will make brief mention of other factors outside cardiovascular conditioning that can influence performance, such as nutrition, strength training, and sports technique. Did you notice the latter two components—strength and technique—are also physical in nature? It just points out the extreme bias that traditional training has toward movement as the only variable worthy of preparation to excel in sport.

Physical training for all sports includes the three fundamentals of traditional training that I've mentioned—cardiovascular conditioning, skill development, and resistance training. All these abilities are critical, and excellent sports performance cannot happen without proficiency in these areas. Depending on your sport and the mindset of your coach (if you have one), you will spend more or less of your training time and energy on these different areas to the point of excluding others, as I did.

It wasn't until I entered collegiate gymnastics with a different coach that I was instructed to run distance as part of my conditioning program. My previous coaches had never incorporated cardiovascular endurance into my workouts. Daily practice only consisted of resistance training, skill development, and repetition of event routines. Likewise, as a mountain bike racer, my coach instructed me to spend most of my time riding my bike, and primarily my road bike for cardiovascular endurance. I wasn't doing any resistance training, and I spent very little time on the technical skills of trail riding or working on my pedaling technique for greater efficiency.

Given that most traditional training plans are biased toward one or two physical areas of training, how can we expect to find consideration for other non-physical factors to balance our athletic performance? We need a new, more wholistic approach to sports training, an approach that doesn't just address only a part of the person, such as the physical body, but instead that prepares the whole person for athletics.

Training the Whole Athlete

Some people are lousy golfers. It's not that the physical mechanics of just hitting a little white (or, in my case, pink) ball are overly demanding (though doing so with accuracy, consistency and appropriate speed and direction require exceptional skill), but rather these people can't master the cognitive aspects of the game. Golf is a highly mental sport. Once you have some proficiency of the basic swing, the mind becomes a dominant force in your score. I have played with golfers who throw clubs, swear often, and constantly berate themselves for bad shots. It's not a good time for anyone.

Yes, golf is a game of skill. However, some of the biggest competencies needed are focus, emotional control, and mental calmness. Although a player may be exquisite in the fundamentals of striking the ball, she will not score well if she cannot control her temper and becomes distracted. Achieving a low golf handicap requires much more than physical prowess with a club and a ball. Not surprisingly, this also applies to endurance sports.

How well are you going to perform in a long-distance event if, say, you're exhausted because you were up all night with a sick child? Are still upset and worried because you received a poor job review from your boss the day before? Feel guilty for taking time away from your family to travel and race without them? Aren't excited to participate and feel like you are being peer pressured into competing? Haven't maintained your equipment or have old gear that you fear may fail? Lack confidence that you can reach your goal of finishing, placing, or winning? Don't have a goal and feel unprepared? Skipped breakfast and have a headache because all you consumed was coffee? Often, few of these factors are considered by athletes who are following the guidance of traditional training. Yet, these factors can all dramatically undermine performance. The results of a competition rest not only on your physical aptitudes, but are also determined by your mental, emotional, and spiritual states.

The athlete cannot be separated from the person. Actually, participation in sports often showcases personality. Instead of a job interview, some companies take a prospective hire out for a round of golf. On the course, away from the office environment, future employers can more easily obtain an accurate read on the personality of the individual they are considering for a job. Here, employers can see how prospective employees will handle themselves in different situations and under stress.[1] They know that you bring your mental, emotional, and moral characteristics with you to sport. If you are anxious, upbeat, tired, grateful, unmotivated, dishonest, or fearful, it will be apparent in how you perform.

The Secret to Peak Performance: Total Alignment

The best athlete is in alignment—physically, mentally, emotionally, and spiritually. This athlete is aligned not just in body as discussed previously, but also in mind and soul. I refer to this as "total alignment." During a victorious performance, an athlete may refer to experiencing "flow" or being in "the zone." Mihaly Csikszentmihalyi, Hungarian psychologist and optimal experience researcher, defines "flow" as follows:

A sense that one's skills are adequate to cope with the challenges at hand, in a goal-directed, rule-bound action system that provides clear clues as to how one is performing. Concentration is so intense that there is no attention left to think about anything irrelevant, or to

training

worry about problems. Self-consciousness disappears, and the sense of time becomes disoriented.[2]

Ursula Grobler, American rower, recalls being in "the zone" during her gold medal performance at the *World Indoor Rowing Championships* in 2010:

Part of the magic of finding and staying in your Zone during competition is that you're no longer competing in your mind. That is, you're not preoccupied with thinking about what you're doing. You've trained enough; your body and muscles know what they're supposed to do. Just let them do it and enjoy the ride, enjoy the game.[3]

I would equate "flow" or "the zone" to being in "total alignment." If you are out of balance in any of these areas, achieving this desired state of performance is elusive. I recall a time when I was in "the zone" on my mountain bike.

It was 2004 during a circuit race in Breckenridge, Colorado. Riding multiple laps on the same course, I recollect going faster and faster each time. It was as if I had become one with the trail. I didn't see any obstacles, only the smooth line before me. My body relaxed and floated effortlessly up and down the dirt path. The crowd disappeared. My mind was calm and focused, completely absorbed in the present. It felt as though I were riding outside myself. I was exhilarated, having no concept of my effort or time passing. When asked why I race, it is for these unforgettable experiences. I don't recall my race result that day, but I'll always treasure the memory of being in "the zone."

In *Zone Mind, Zone Body*, Roy Palmer, Alexander Technique® teacher and sports coach, defines seven characteristics of "the zone" experience that reflect "total alignment":

(1) Being totally absorbed and focused on the activity. (2) Experience of an internal clarity and understanding exactly what is required, knowing their skills are matched to the task. (3) A sense of ecstasy—

being outside everyday reality. (4) "Being in the moment" focusing completely on the present. Unaware of time passing—a sense of time slowing down. (5) A deep passion for the activity leading to higher levels of performance. (6) Sense of serenity—no anxiety, no ego, no worries about the outcome of action. (7) No sense of effort. The activity becomes easy. Getting out of the way.[4]

These seven characteristics tie together your personal traits in the four dimensions—physical, mental, emotional, and spiritual. When all these aspects are balanced, you can reach peak performance. Jim Loehr and Tony Schwartz, leaders in human performance, cite harmony in these same areas as necessary for full engagement: "To be fully engaged, you must be physically energized, emotionally connected, mentally focused and spiritually aligned with a purpose beyond our immediate self-interest."[5]

When fully engaged, you can reach the Ideal Performance State (IPS). In the book, *The New Toughness Training for Sports*, Loehr defines IPS:

> The optimal state of physiological and psychological arousal for performing at your peak. [...] You are most likely to experience IPS and perform at your peak when you feel: confident, relaxed and calm, energized with positive emotion, challenged, focused and alert, automatic and instinctive, ready for fun and enjoyment.[6]

Regardless of the name—"flow," "the zone," "full engagement," or "IPS"—the meaning is the same. You are aligned in the four critical dimensions—physically, mentally, emotionally, and spiritually. In my opinion, this "total alignment" is at the center of athletic success, as you will see in my model for sports performance.

Wheel of Sports Performance

While studying to become a wellness coach, I was introduced to the "Wheel of Life" in Michael Arloski's book, *Wellness Coaching for Lasting Lifestyle Change*.[7] This is a pie-chart model used to help people identify where they are doing well and where there is room for improvement in various facets of their lives. There are many versions of the wheel of life,

training

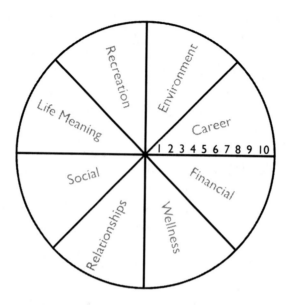

Figure 13-1. The Wheel of Life assesses balance between the different areas of your life.

most with six to eight sections depicted. I have made my own model by combining several commonly used concepts, just to give you the idea (Figure 13-1). My sample Wheel of Life includes environment, career, financial, wellness, relationships, social, life meaning, and recreation.

To use the Wheel of Life, a person rates his satisfaction level in each section of the wheel from 1 (lowest) in the center of the wheel to 10 (highest) on the outer edge of the wheel for each of the eight sections. Upon examination of the results, it is common to find some sections that are high, and others that are low or totally neglected. The diagram raises your understanding about the diversity of life and is used to assess life balance. It creates recognition about what is deficient, which can inspire action for positive change.

Applying this tool to wholistic sports training, I identified six components essential for excellence in athletics and developed the "Wheel of Sports Performance." In addition to having six equal sections, my bicycle wheel model has a central piece integrating with and influencing all the others. This essential, connecting piece is "total alignment." It acts as the hub of the wheel (Figure 13-2). Without a hub, the wheel cannot roll, loses

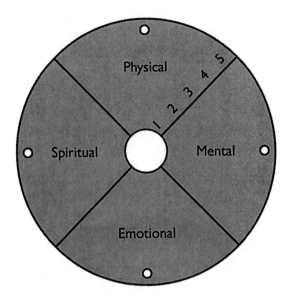

Figure 13-2. The hub of the Wheel of Sports Performance contains the four dimensions of "total alignment"—physical, mental, emotional, and spiritual.

integrity, and falls apart. The flexible, wired spokes of a bicycle wheel connect the hub to the rim and give the wheel its shape. If the wheel has no hub, the spokes have no internal attachment and will quickly fail.

I have talked a great deal about physical alignment as it relates to your body structure and biomechanics. It is the base of the Sports Training Pyramid in Chapter 12. But what does it mean to be aligned in the other dimensions? Using Loehr and Schwartz's model of "full engagement", I've listed a few of the traits given for each area. Emotionally, you are confident, in control, and trusting. Mentally, you are having a good time, are prepared, and express creativity. Spiritually, you exhibit honesty, courage, and commitment.[5] Using these descriptions as well as your own interpretation of these dimensions, think about how you would score on a scale of 1-5, 1 being the lowest and 5 being the highest. You'll have an opportunity to complete the model at the end of the chapter.

In my pie-chart model, each of the six slices in the spoke area of the wheel that surrounds the hub represents a section that is pertinent to top sports performance. The hub is the foundation of these attributes, which radiate out to the rim. Surrounding the inner hub of the wheel are the

training

symmetrical sections of (1) sports fitness, (2) supportive environment, (3) health conditions, (4) body composition, (5) nutrition, and (6) strategy (Figure 13-3). I will introduce each section and provide guidance, without going into great detail. Please note that I am not writing a cookie-cutter training book with a stepwise approach or in-depth workout descriptions. There are already plenty of those available lining my book shelves, and maybe yours, too. Rather, my goal in this chapter is to introduce you to the components of a wholistic training program.

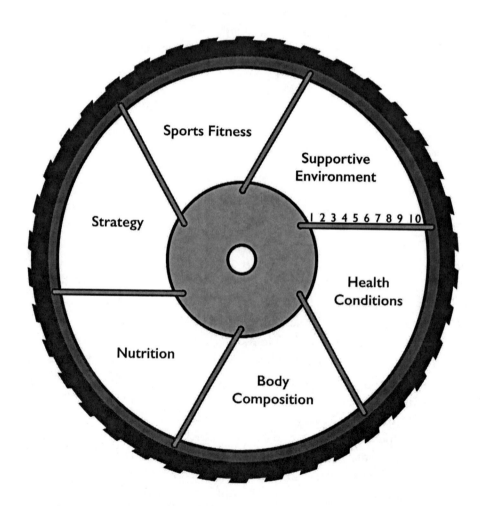

Figure 13-3. The spoke area of the Wheel of Sports Performance contains six equally sized sections, all of which influence your athletics.

1. Sports Fitness

Cardiovascular conditioning, skills development, and resistance training constitute the three elements of sports fitness as discussed in the traditional training approach at the beginning of this chapter. Every athlete needs to incorporate all three areas of fitness, although the percentage of emphasis will vary in accordance with the demands of the sport, specifics of the peak event, and strengths and weaknesses of the individual athlete.

Cardiovascular conditioning targets the heart and circulatory system. This system provides the body with essential nutrients, including oxygen, while also removing metabolic waste products, such as lactate. Three energy systems are built with cardiovascular conditioning: (1) the short-acting phosphagen system for maximal efforts of 10 seconds or less; (2) the anaerobic (without oxygen) system, also referred to as glycolysis, for athletic pursuits of 30 seconds to two minutes; and (3) the aerobic (with oxygen) system, providing sustained energy for long durations (anything over two minutes).[8]

Depending on the demands of your sport and your personal strengths and weaknesses, your training emphasizes these different energy systems at varying degrees. For example, a sprinter focuses many workouts on the phosphagen system with repeated efforts of 10 seconds or less. A long-distance athlete like myself will prioritize building the aerobic energy system, within which are several levels, including lactate threshold, VO_2max, tempo, and more. As a self-coached athlete for most of my career, I found Joe Friel's series of *Training Bibles*[9] easy to follow, with good progressions and a variety of workouts.

Skill development can take many forms—sports-specific tricks, flexibility, speed, power, agility—whatever assets are required for successful performance. Examples include vertical jump, tennis serve, volleyball dig, throwing, etc. A skill I have had to work on is flat, powerful riding. Being small and living in a hilly environment, I am a decent climber, but I am slow and quickly fatigue on the steady, flat grades. By the way, notice that I have purposely not included the word "technique" in reference to skill; I will talk about that in detail in Chapter 14.

Resistance training pushes the musculoskeletal and neuromuscular systems to overcome a load. This was thoroughly discussed in Chapter 12. Another variable that you can change, though, and one that I often practice,

training

is adding resistance to the training surface. Examples include running or biking on trails, since sand or gravel provides more resistance than a paved road; playing tennis on grass or clay rather than a hard court; roller skiing on asphalt with the speed reducers engaged; or simply going uphill in any form—hike, bike, etc.

Sports-specific resistance can also be applied. Strap on a parachute during a track workout; put a resistance band around your midsection and have your training partner maintain tension while you run or bound uphill; practice your golf swing with a weighted club; wear multiple swimsuits to create drag in the pool; or use the higher gears on your bike. Once you reduce the resistance, you'll find you can move much easier and with less effort.

2. Supportive Environment

It's tough to be a Nordic skier in the southwest, which is why I would spend my winters in Hailey, Idaho, whenever possible. While there, I had access to world-renowned ski trails, fabulous fitness facilities, numerous top-rated exercise classes, and a large community of enthusiastic skiers. Prior to this luxury, I skied and raced competitively while living in Los Alamos, New Mexico, spending many hours roller skiing on the roads to mimic the skiing movements and resistance of snow.

A prospective coach once told me I needed to move to Boulder, Colorado, where the weather is more mild, if I wanted to take my mountain bike racing seriously. Needless to say, I didn't hire him. The outdoor temperature of where you live is only one consideration in your environment. There are many other factors that can equally affect your training. Even when you can't get outdoors, effective training can happen if you have the appropriate support and resources.

A supportive environment starts at home. Does your significant other support your athletics or try to sabotage your training? Is your partner health conscious like you, or does he prepare high-fat meals, make tempting desserts, and encourage alcohol consumption? Do you train with members of your family, or do you feel rushed to get back to them? I am lucky in this respect: my husband is also a competitor, so we share similar lifestyle values. When one of us wants to be lazy and skip a workout, the other is there with an encouraging word.

It can be hard when you have a family. There are more responsibilities and demands on your time. I know of couples who alternate years or seasons in their competitive aspirations. One year or season is her turn, and the next is his. She may run races in the warmer months, while he ski races in the winter, or vice versa. They support each other in their sports while balancing the needs of the family.

Work can also get in the way of training. How my clients joke about this! Do you have a supportive boss who lets you come in a little later to fit in a morning training session, take extra time at lunch, or leave a bit early for your evening group workout? At the height of my professional mountain biking career, I was able to drop down to part-time at my job to accommodate a higher training load.

Your gear is also part of your environment. Do you have appropriate and up-to-date toys? Is everything in working order? From experience, I know that leaking goggles can ruin your swim workout! Is your equipment easily accessible? Having my bike trainer already set up in the house makes it a lot more inviting to ride.

If the weather does turn bad, do you have appropriate clothing to exercise in colder temperatures? Being prepared with suitable gear—and having a backup plan, such as going to the gym, if it's just too terrible outside—are essential components of a supportive environment.

3. Health Conditions

Health conditions aside from injury and pain, such as headaches, high blood pressure or cholesterol, irritable bowel syndrome, insomnia, anxiety disorders, and others, need to be in control to enable your best performance. Several famous athletes have overcome their health conditions to achieve greatness in sport. Kris Freeman, Nordic Olympian and veteran of the U.S. Ski Team, has successfully managed Type 1 diabetes for over a decade by collaborating with gifted endocrinologists.[10] Wilma Rudolph, a track and field athlete, overcame polio as a child to win three gold medals in the *1960 Summer Olympic Games*.[11] Amy Van Dyken, six-time Olympic gold medalist in swimming, suffered from severe asthma and couldn't even swim the length of the pool when she started at the age of six.[12] Jason Day, Australian professional golfer and tour member, collapsed on the golf course

training

with vertigo in the summer of 2015,[13] only to be ranked first in the world in March of 2016.[14]

Health conditions do not have to hamper your sports, but they do have to be considered and controlled. If you are living with a chronic health condition, or if you experience occasional illness such as seasonal allergies or menstrual cramps, seek the appropriate treatment to keep yourself healthy and able to train and compete.

4. Body Composition

You can be a good athlete regardless of your size and weight! Optimizing your body composition, however, can improve your performance and reduce your risk of injury.

Body efficiency is your ability to convert chemical energy—food—into mechanical energy—physical output. The efficiency of the human body can be measured either by strength-to-weight ratio (SWR) or by body composition. Your SWR is calculated by dividing your weight by your strength, as determined in the weight room. The lower your mass and the more force you can produce, the fitter you are and the more you'll be able to do before reaching fatigue.[15] For instance, if you can squat 150 pounds and you weigh 150 pounds, your SWR is 1, which is considered good. If, however, your weight were 125 pounds, your SWR would be 1.2, even better. The higher your ratio, the greater your efficiency.[15]

Body composition testing, the other method for measuring efficiency, gives you insight into the makeup of your body mass so you'll know how much of you is fat and how much of you is fat-free mass. A standard scale is blind and cannot give you such distinctions. For example, a scale only displays that you weigh 140 pounds; body composition testing can break that down into 40 pounds of fat and 100 pounds of fat-free mass. If you lose fat and gain muscle—which weighs more than fat—the numbers on the scale may not change, or they could go up, which can be quite discouraging. The real story of what is happening within your body can be observed through body composition testing. Through this testing, you might find that although your overall weight didn't change, you lowered your fat mass to 35 pounds and increased your fat-free mass to 105 pounds. Your strength and efficiency are greater even though the number on the scale stayed the same.

Body composition is measured by various techniques. Two of the most accessible and least expensive are skinfolds and bioelectrical impedance. Assessing skin folds requires pinching and measuring your subcutaneous (under the skin) fat in specific areas of the body. For reliable measurements and consistency, a trained technician is essential. If you have this test performed at your local health club, make sure you have the same person do it each time. Also ensure that your body is in the same state each time regarding prior exercise and hydration level. You can also do the test at home yourself by purchasing a set of calipers.

Measuring body composition with bioelectrical impedance can be as easy as standing on a scale hooked up with monitoring sensors. Bioelectrical impedance sends an electrical current through your tissues and measures the speed of transmission. A faster current equates to more fat-free mass. Like the skinfold readings, make sure your body is in the same state each time you use the scale. Transmission of the current is highly affected by the amount of water in your tissues.

Although both techniques are convenient and relatively inexpensive, they are also the least accurate, with a 3-5 percent error rate.[16] If you are most interested in tracking changes in body fat and are okay having some error in the actual number, these are good choices. If you'd prefer more accurate numbers, you'll want to seek out one of the following more precise techniques: underwater weighing—comparing your normal body weight and underwater weight; the Bod Pod—measuring air displacement in a sealed chamber; or a Dual-Energy X-Ray Absorptiometry (DEXA) scan. These tests give you more exact body composition numbers, but they will also hit your pocketbook harder and may not be available in your community.

Even though a high percentage of fat-free mass is desirable and increases your strength-to-weight ratio, an essential amount of fat is necessary for survival. Too little body fat can impair your health and your performance. The American College of Sports Medicine (ACSM) recommends a minimum of 3 percent fat for men and 12 percent fat for women.[17] According to the ACSM, when we drop below these fat percentages, the body is negatively impacted in such necessary functions as "delivery of vitamins to the organs, the ability of the reproductive system to function, and overall well-being."[17]

The ACSM considers 10-22 percent fat healthy for men and 20-32 percent fat healthy for women.[17] You can find further breakdowns of body fat ranges for various sports and ages on the internet. Since these measure-

training

ments vary widely and are likely to change, I have not listed any resources here. I also don't want you to become obsessed with the numbers. Rather, tune in to how you feel and function at different body weights. You'll tend to find there is a range at which you are strongest and a level below which you should not go.

If body composition is holding you back from attaining your athletic potential, consider consulting with a registered dietitian who specializes in sports nutrition and possibly body image concerns.

Weight and body size have been ongoing issues for me. Not that I'm big, but as a gymnast, I could never be slim enough. Daily weigh-ins on a standard scale and being regularly berated by my coach about my figure have left scars in my mind. I recall my teammates coming to my defense—I was the skinniest one—but it was of no use. I would never be light enough. Many of my teammates had weight issues of their own, and a few succumbed to eating disorders. I tried crazy diets, too, but none for long. I just could not survive a four-hour gymnastics workout on grapefruit alone.

Weight loss is a complicated issue with multiple factors. If this is your key objective, you'll want to ensure you are losing fat while maintaining your fat-free mass. Additionally, you might also need to address any deeper issues that are preventing you from reaching and maintaining your ideal weight. From my experience with clients, there is often a mental and emotional aspect to weight control that can impede progress, making goals unattainable by solely cutting calories or increasing activity.

5. Nutrition

Closely related to body composition are your dietary practices. *Food is fuel!* The quality and quantity of what you put into your body will impact your sports performance. Is your body responding well to what you are putting in your engine? I have seen clients experience dramatic improvements after making dietary changes—abstaining from gluten and/or dairy, eating more raw unprocessed foods, increasing anti-inflammatory foods, changing body pH, and significantly increasing hydration.

Eating well takes planning. You likely follow a training plan for your athletic workouts. The same amount of careful consideration should be given to the foods supporting your efforts—meals, snacks, and pre-during-post workout nutrition. Timing of healthy foods is also critical to ensure consistent energy without hitting the wall (depleting your energy reserves) during exercise, which results in a rapid deterioration in performance.

The composition of your diet matters. Nancy Clark, M.S., R.D., C.S.S.D., internationally recognized sports nutritionist and bestselling author, recommends that the base of an athlete's calories comes from carbohydrates—vegetables, whole grains, fruit, beans and dairy.[18] Carbohydrates are the primary fuel source for aerobic exercise. Fats also propel us during long-distance exercise and should comprise a quarter or more of our intake. The more intense the exercise effort, however, the higher the percentage of carbohydrates used. Protein, which helps build muscle and repair tissue, is only used as a fuel source when the others are lacking. Intake of protein should be less than the other two nutrients, about 10-15 percent.[18] This is only very basic sports nutrition information. For more guidance on good sources of carbohydrates, proteins and fats, what to eat and when, menu suggestions, and lots of great recipes, check out *Nancy Clark's Sports Nutrition Guidebook.*[18]

One of the best ways to evaluate your diet is through daily recording. Start by documenting everything you eat for three days. Next, plug the information into one of the many dietary analysis tools available online. At the time of this writing, myfitnesspal, www.myfitnesspal.com, was one of the top-rated food and nutrition tracking online tools. Generally, these online trackers provide reports with breakdowns of each nutrient category, as well as recommendations for dietary changes.

6. Strategy

Strategy, the final section of the Wheel of Sports Performance, crosses many training aspects. In fact, I've already talked about a strategy for each of the prior five slices in the model. Since there are so many areas I'd like to address regarding strategy, I'm devoting Chapter 14 to the new approaches I've developed after my injuries.

Before I move on to the new strategies, though, I'd like to take a few moments to discuss some well-known and tested strategies that are still

training

applicable and important for sports excellence. In Chapter 3, I recommended setting recovery goals. Since I am an advocate of focusing your training toward your highest priority event, I strongly recommend setting goals for your sports season. These goals should include more than just winning or placing in competition. There should also be specific performance objectives, such as learning an advanced skill, meeting a time goal in practice, or improving in any of the categories previously discussed.

Periodization, which means dividing your training up into phases, is another fundamental concept in peak sports performance. You can't train hard all the time, and if you don't put in the exhaustive efforts at the right time, you won't be in the best shape for your event. Doing the correct workouts at the correct time is imperative to reaching your goals. My husband refers to this as making deposits in your training bank that you'll withdraw from during competition. To perform well, you'll need to build up your reserves. The year can be split up into phases—preparation, build, peak, transition—to maximize your sports season performance. For more guidance on periodization, I again refer you to one of Joe Friel's books in his *Training Bible* series.[9]

Within the strategy of periodization is the concept of gradual progression. Friel recommends increasing annual hours by 10-15 percent.[9] You can extrapolate this out to only increasing your workload by that small percentage week to week, while scheduling in a recovery week every four to six weeks. For example, if your average training is 10 hours a week, a conservative increase of approximately 10 percent a week over a five-week block would be the following: 11 hours the first week, 12 hours the second week, 13 hours the third week and 14 hours the fourth week, followed by a light recovery week of 5-7 hours.

Tactics are an additional element to consider for your event. You'll need a plan about when to exert your effort and when to hold back. Sometimes the risk of falling while bombing a downhill section of trail on bike, foot, or skis is not worth the possible minimal time gains. You might also have to determine your tactics about how and when you can eat during your event. It can be tough to eat during some events like a mountain bike race. When I pre-ride the course before a race, I figure out what sections are best suited for taking in calories. I often fill a flask with energy gel and mount it to my bike; that way, I can quickly grab the flask at the most opportune time.

You'll also need to be prepared for pre-event anxiety. What are the butterflies in your stomach telling you? Well, it depends on your interpretation. Do you recognize the butterflies to be a sign that you are fearful, not prepared, and doubtful of your fitness? Or do you view the butterflies as an indication that you are excited, ready, and confident? How you interpret your physical sensations and what words you tell yourself greatly influence your anxiety level. Strive to be calm. Develop pre-event rituals such as listening to music, minimizing your exposure to the nervous energy of others, or breathing deeply. For example, so that I don't get distracted, stressed, or sucked into the anxious starting line chatter, I only come up to the line right before the gun goes off.

You'll learn more strategies in Chapter 14. But now let's move on to using the Wheel of Sports Performance.

Using the Wheel of Sports Performance

The Wheel of Sports Performance evaluates your personal and sports training balance. The tire surrounding the outside of the wheel needs to be fully inflated, operating at a high pressure, to perform optimally. If one or more of your wheel slices is not well practiced, lacks mastery, and is under-inflated, you're in for a bumpy ride. Your wheel will only roll smoothly if you are in "total alignment" and equally proficient in all the training sections of the wheel.

In my model, each area of the wheel is given the same parameters because all are equally valuable. Just one low-scoring section can increase your susceptibility to injury and pain. Ratings, 1 (lowest) in the center of the wheel to 10 (highest) on the outer edge of the wheel, like those on the Wheel of Life, are based on your level of satisfaction and competence in each area. Recall that the inner hub has a rating scale of 1 to 5.

Before my injuries, I did not have this model to use and could not assess where I was out of balance in my "total alignment" and sports training. I wish I had so that I could have avoided some of the mistakes I repeatedly made. Upon reflection, my wheel would have looked like the image in Figure 13-4.

Viewing this graphic as a true bike wheel along the outer edge, it is apparent that I was in for a jarring ride. None of my scores reached the edge

training

Hub		Spoke Area	
Physical	1	Sports Fitness	5
Mental	3	Supportive Environment	8
Emotional	4	Health Conditions	4
Spiritual	2	Body Composition	7
		Nutrition	6
		Strategy	3

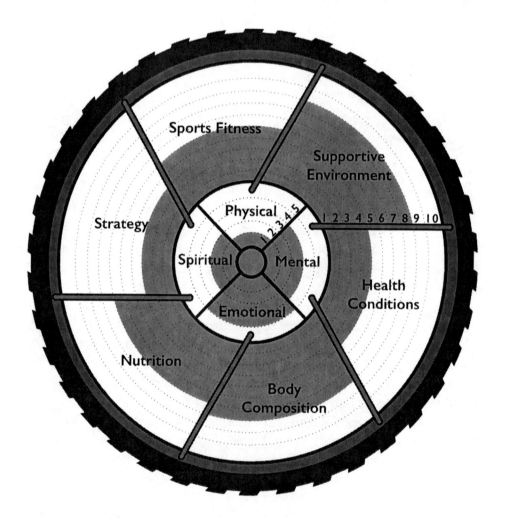

Figure 13-4. A depiction of what my Wheel of Sports Performance would have looked like before my injuries and chronic pain.

of the wheel. Although I was close in some areas, I had lots of work to do in others. Wheel balance is disrupted when the sections are unevenly weighted. You'll feel a noticeable "thunk" with every revolution of the wobbly tire. Additionally, I would have been lucky if my wheel held together at all with its lack of integrity at the inner hub. The goal for all of us is to flow easily down our path.

Your Wheel of Sports Performance

How smooth does your wheel roll? Use the Wheel of Sports Performance to find out (Figure 13-5). Make copies of the assessment on the following two pages to use over and over at different time intervals—one month, four months, one year—to measure your progress toward balanced training. You can also download additional copies of the Wheel of Sports Performance from my website, www.thepfathlete.com/resources. Viewing your wheel will help you see where the gaps are in your training, and it could help you to determine which deficiencies may have been contributing factors to your injury. As you return to sport using this tool, you can adopt a more wholistic approach to your sports preparation.

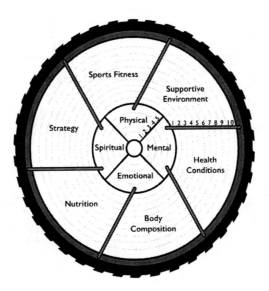

Figure 13-5. The Wheel of Sports Performance assesses balance between the different components of sports training.

training

Wheel of Sports Performance

Fill in the Wheel of Sports Performance with your number ratings and color in the corresponding area. The resulting image will give you a picture of your training balance. To assess each area in the Wheel of Sports Performance, consider the following questions.

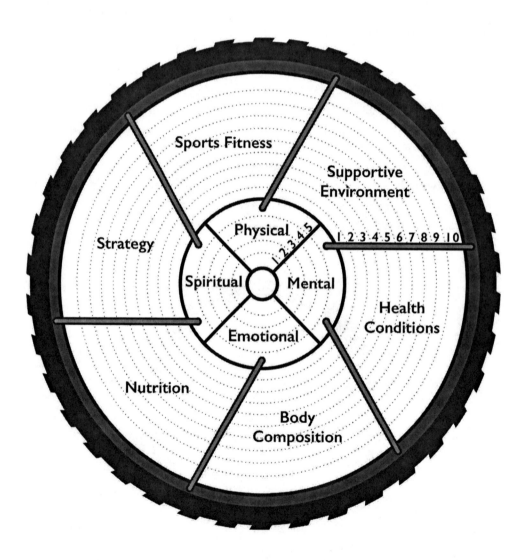

The Hub—Total Alignment

Physical Alignment: *Is your skeletal position balanced? Are your muscles and joints functioning efficiently without dysfunctions and compensations?*

Mental Alignment: *Do you have an optimistic mindset, free from excess stress? Are you at peace, calm, focused, and expressing creativity?*

Emotional Alignment: *Are you experiencing joy, love, and connection with others? Are you accepting today? Do you feel hopeful for the future?*

Spiritual Alignment: *Are you living your values, expressing yourself authentically, and finding deeper meaning or a sense of purpose in life?*

Outer Wheel

Sports Fitness: *Do you have the cardiovascular fitness, sports skills, and physical strength needed to excel in your sport?*

Supportive Environment: *Does your physical and social environment provide safety, encouragement and opportunity for your sports participation?*

Health Conditions: *Are you managing your health conditions and not allowing them to control or limit your training and competition?*

Body Composition: *Do you have a good strength-to-weight ratio and/or percentage of body fat in the desirable range?*

Nutrition: *Are you using food as fuel for your sport, proportioning your nutrient calories appropriately for your workouts and making healthy eating choices?*

Strategy: *Do you have a strategy for all the factors that can influence your performance and results?*

training

Summary

Exceptional sports performance requires more than physical prowess alone. Great athletes experience "flow" or being in "the zone" during extraordinary achievements. This is a cognitive state of clarity, ease, mindfulness, focus, and serenity. "Flow" or "the zone" is entered when you, the athlete, are in harmony and are optimally functioning physically, mentally, emotionally, and spiritually. These four dimensions of "total alignment" form the hub of my Wheel of Sports Performance. This model is a guide for wholistic training. The model includes additional variables that are frequently neglected in traditional sports training, which has been heavily focused only on conditioning the body physically. Surrounding the inner hub of the model are six equal wheel sections—(1) sports fitness, (2) supportive environment, (3) health conditions, (4) body composition, (5) nutrition and (6) strategy.

Just like your body needs a strong core at your center, your training and performance requires a sturdy hub. Otherwise, like the sandcastle, which lacks internal support, you may struggle in reaching your sports goals. A well-balanced wheel is achieved when all the areas are weighted evenly. Adopting a wholistic approach to training will provide you with a smooth ride to athletic excellence.

Game Winning Strategies

1. <u>Complete the Wheel of Sports Performance</u>

Take time to honestly assess where you rate in each of the areas on the wheel. After you do, put the model away for a day or so. Then re-check your numbers and choose one area you'd like to target for improvement. Start with one easy step you can do right away to raise your score in that section. Once accomplished, build in that same area or pick another slice for advancement. Keep your steps small but steady.

To repeat the assessment and track your progress, you can download additional copies of the Wheel of Sports Performance from my website, www.thepfathlete.com/resources.

2. <u>Balance Your Wheel With Coaching</u>

If you found your Wheel of Sports Performance or Wheel of Life was lopsided, consider partnering with a coach. A coach can provide support, accountability and guidance to assist you in reaching your health, athletic, and life goals. A balanced training program helps prevent future injuries and pain. Learn more about coaching with The Pain Free Athlete: www.thepfathlete.com.

3. <u>Document a Flow Experience</u>

Recall a time when you were in "flow," "the zone," "full engagement," or the "ideal performance state." It could be during sports but doesn't have to be. Write as much as you can about the experience, as many details as you can remember. *What were you sensing—physically, mentally, emotionally, and spiritually?* This "total alignment" is the basis of optimal sports performance, the hub of your Wheel of Sports Performance. Reflect on this time in your life. Balancing your wheel will build more of these positive, joyful memories.

training

14

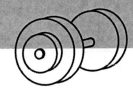

Seven Strategies for Sports Performance

*T*he idea of "respect" is the underlying theme of my strategies for sports training and performance. Through my healing process, I learned appreciation and gratitude for activity. I became more connected with my body and developed a deeper understanding of its needs. I committed to no longer taking my structure for granted; I dedicated myself to stop inflicting endless abuse while ignoring my body's warnings. Upon my recovery, I was determined to train and compete without pain and further body destruction. What follows are seven of the new strategies I implemented to reach this goal. I encourage you to consider them as you re-enter or continue in sports.

Strategy 1: Have a Flexible Plan

As a professional athlete, I was a slave to my daily training plan and my "Sports Gremlin." I modeled the term Sports Gremlin after the depiction of our negative inner critic from Rick Carson's acclaimed book, *Taming Your Gremlin*®.[1] Carson, who is a coach, trainer, author and founder of the Gremlin-Taming® Institute,[2] refers to this negative inner critic this way:

> A Gremlin in your head and he's out to make you miserable. Left to do his thing, he'll zap your health, foul up your relationships, ruin your disposition, dampen your creativity, hamper your productivity, drive you into low-down funks and wind you up into fits of anxiety.[2]

Your Sports Gremlin is specific to your athletic life. This is the voice of the unrelenting taskmaster inside that makes darn sure you stick to your training plan—no matter what. Your Sports Gremlin scares you into making bad choices that are self-destructive for your body and soul. In my case, I had to adhere dutifully to my training plan, lest my Sports Gremlin would start shrieking at me.

In the past, my Sports Gremlin didn't let me rest. He encouraged me to push through pain, regardless of the consequences. You'll notice I referred to my Sports Gremlin as a "he." Since most of my coaches were men, my Sports Gremlin was a male, but yours may be a woman. Subconsciously, I chose to give him power and control over my actions. My Sports Gremlin urged me to train constantly, harder and longer than my competitors—train until I couldn't train anymore, and then dig deeper to keep going. My Sports Gremlin warned that I'd get fat and lose fitness if I took a day off. Do you know this voice? Your Sports Gremlin may have a tone similar to mine.

For example, my Sports Gremlin said, "Even though my knee hurts, I have to do my intervals today. That's the plan. I can't do them tomorrow anyway. It's my most important workout of the week, and if I don't do them right now, my training plan is shot. The race is only three weeks away. I need to get fitter if I want to be on the podium. Don't be a wimp, take a painkiller and get to work!"

I wrote this in the first person because your Sports Gremlin is a part of you. My Sports Gremlin was definitely a part of me, something I had created. It is difficult for anyone to say *NO* to their Sports Gremlin.

One summer during the competitive season, I had been traveling to mountain bike races every weekend. I was exhausted and didn't want to go on the road again. I needed a break. The result? My Sports Gremlin threw a hissy fit. He tried to bully and intimidate me into doing what he wanted. Sports Gremlins vigorously fight change. They don't have your best interests in mind and are intent on making you suffer.[2] Fortunately, I talked to my coach, who didn't agree with my Sports Gremlin. I took the weekend off, but it was very hard. It felt like failure.

Once you are aware of your Sports Gremlin and the tactics he uses to get you to do what he wants, you are empowered. You can make a choice to buy into the illogical and harmful advice, or you can just observe. Instead of jumping to your Sports Gremlin's commands, you can sit back and watch his antics. After witnessing his desperate show, you can make a mindful choice to act or not. It is this separation and external perspective that allows you to make better decisions. When you do this, you take away your Sports Gremlin's power, and his voice fades. This is one of the lessons of Gremlin-Taming®.[2]

With your Sports Gremlin in check, you can make more intelligent and respectful choices about your training. Some days you just don't feel up to it for a variety of reasons—and that's okay. Now, instead of having a daily training plan, I have a more flexible week plan. I list out the workouts and give them a priority. When I feel good, I do my highest priority training, and when I don't, I do something more moderate, or I rest. This is less stressful; it allows me more control. This way, I get the most out of each workout. I don't feel pressured to push myself on days I don't have the energy—physically, mentally, emotionally, or spiritually. A great deal of an effective workout comes down to your attitude and willingness to go beyond what is comfortable. Some days I embrace that challenge, and some days I can't face it. If you start to have too many days where you're not motivated for your sports training, you might need to look at other life factors, such as your daily stress level.

Strategy 2: Balance Stress and Recovery

An essential component of a flexible training plan is adequate rest and recovery. When I talk about rest, I am referring to more than sleep. Of course, sound sleep is essential for continued sports training. The body assimilates all the work you've done throughout the day when you are asleep. The body regenerates while you slumber. Most athletes don't have much trouble sleeping: a tough workout is an antidote for sleeplessness. However, many athletes do have trouble resting and taking time off from their sport.

Fitness is gained when you rest! Your workouts break your body down. It is commonly accepted that you don't weight train the same muscles every day because you would continually grow weaker with each workout. Every

303

time you lift weights, micro-tears are created in your muscles. Adequate rest is needed to allow the muscles to repair themselves and grow stronger. Without this essential recovery time, the muscles would be repeatedly broken down and would weaken.[3] The same principle applies to endurance sports. You are depleting your body with each hill you climb and interval you complete. The body can only grow to a stronger, fitter state if it's allowed the time and rest it needs to rebuild. Often a night of sleep is not enough for you to fully recover. Knowing this, many training plans encourage one or two days of rest each week. The challenge is getting you, the athlete, to follow this advice.

Rest can be active or passive. "Active rest" means working out with very low intensity. If you are a runner, you'd walk or hike. "Passive rest" is refraining from all activity, not doing any exercise. It can be hard for a motivated athlete to keep her effort low enough during active rest, which is why I often recommend passive rest. While the mind has a hard time with passive rest, it is just what the body craves.

Marvin Zauderer, MFT, coach and psychotherapist, explains that our inability to rest hinges on our desire to be in control:

> In Western culture, we tend to be consumed by the perspective that the thing that we want to happen—getting stronger, faster, fitter—is happening only when we're working on it, exerting some kind of control. We aren't used to the idea that letting go, resting and relaxing control can be as important to healing recovery, and strengthening as they are.[4]

We mistakenly believe that we need to be actively engaging in our sport to gain fitness when actually the opposite is true. In reality, to become better athletes, we need to let go of the constant activity and striving. We need to schedule rest and downtime into our training plans. We need to balance the stress of training and life; we must relax and let the body achieve gains through stillness.

I recall talking to a fellow professional mountain biker about her training one season. She told me she wasn't doing any intervals and was keeping her rides at a lower, though challenging, intensity and was resting more. I was astonished! I thought we had to up

our training efforts every year. More shocking, however, was her renewed fitness and drive to compete. She was having the best race results of her career, beating competitors that were previously beyond her wheels.

Unfortunately, many of us tend to adhere to the demands of our Sports Gremlin, and we continue working to maintain control. We push our bodies to the brink of collapse, injury or sickness rather than taking a rest day to recover and grow stronger. Achieving athletic goals was paramount to everything else for my client, Trish.

Trish is an exceptional athlete. She excels in road cycling, marathon running, mountain climbing, duathlon, cross-country skiing, and mountain biking. Her athletic accomplishments include qualifying for the *Boston Marathon*, winning numerous hill climb events, placing third in the *United States National Time Trial Championships*, ascending many 13- and 14-thousand-foot peaks in Colorado, coming in fourth in the *USA Triathlon Duathlon National Championships* to qualify for worlds, and achieving a podium finish in a 50-mile mountain bike race.

These athletic achievements came with a cost. Being a multi-sport athlete, Trish never had an offseason, going from training for one event to the next. She was afraid to take a day off, fearing she'd lose fitness and wouldn't be able to get going again. Instead, her philosophy was, "Push as hard as you can all the time, thinking that would make me stronger instead of actually tearing my body down and not being able to repair itself." She recovered by climbing hills at a slightly slower pace.

Even when she knew she was overtrained because her legs and muscles were fatigued and couldn't produce any intensity, she kept going. She saw this as weakness: "I got mad at myself. I wanted to be able to go hard all the time." She saw herself as a failure and disappointment to herself and those around her when she wasn't in top form.

Divorce, injury, and having kids all began to interfere with Trish's training. She would race until she couldn't walk; her left side would go numb in training; and she had searing pain in her back

training

and sacroiliac joints (SIJ). Her motto was "Train through the pain." Highly driven, she continued toward her goals: "I didn't want this injury to get in the way of completing what I was going to do that year. If I say I'm going to do something I'm going to do it, even if I'm limping through it."

Trish finally woke up to her self-destructive pattern after having to take multiple trips to the emergency room, losing weight to the point of being 15 pounds below her ideal weight, and being continuously sick due to inadequate sleep as a new mom with two infants and training for a half marathon. "I had depleted myself and kept going and going. I just got worn out, and my brain finally said, 'You're done. You're burned out. This is it. You've hit the bottom. You have to rest. You have to rest.'"

Like Trish, I didn't value rest. Having surgery or being ill was the only time off I ever afforded myself. It wasn't until I read the article "The Making of a Corporate Athlete"[5] by Jim Loehr and Tony Schwartz, leaders in human performance, that I began to understand the importance of rest. I mentioned this article in the introduction regarding the four energy capacities: physical—ability to do work; mental—cognitive; emotional—inner climate; and spiritual—values and purpose. Exercise is physical stress. You may not think of it this way because it helps you to manage psychological stress, but pushing your body physically is also a form of stress, which can lead to abuse.

The body doesn't distinguish the source of your stress. It is ignorant of why you are experiencing stress, whether it's from a hard workout, fight with a family member, work deadline, traffic jam, or lack of sleep. It just feels the effects of repeated activation of the stress response. But you can only handle so much stress in your life at one time until you deplete your capacities and must recover.

The physical stress of exercise and competition can overwhelm your system when you're already under high stress in other capacities.

Upon losing my beloved dog Coral, I experienced tremendous emotional and mental stress. I was also taxed by a sudden lack of identity and purpose: I was no longer a dog mom, and I no longer had the purpose of rehabbing my canine. Although I had planned to do a race just a few days later, there was NO WAY I could compete. I was completely drained from my loss. My psychological stress was already so great that I couldn't possibly muster the physical energy needed to perform. This is a normal and expected response, regardless of the stress. It is your body's way of helping you slow down and not push yourself to the point of injury or illness.

According to Loehr and Schwartz, the fluid movement between stress and recovery is essential for high performance: "Chronic stress without recovery depletes energy reserves, leads to burnout and breakdown, and ultimately undermines performance."[5] Their premise is that energy, not time, is your most precious resource. And your supply of energy is limited and must be regularly restored in all four capacities—physical, emotional, mental, and spiritual. Rest and recovery rituals renew your energy supply.[5]

To stay healthy, Trish has expanded her recovery rituals from a monthly massage to include regular acupuncture, chiropractic, counseling, and wellness coaching. She also meditates daily and practices yoga and alignment exercises consistently. In describing her need for rest, Trish uses this analogy: "A car has a gas tank, and if you don't refill it, it's not going to go anymore." You need to replenish your energy supplies, which are emptied by stress, so you can continue to train and compete in sports. *This is why you must rest and recover!* I now savor my rest days. *Aaaah!*

Strategy 3: Refine Sports Technique

All sports have an element of technique. Lifting a barbell, pedaling a bicycle, landing a somersault, carving a giant slalom turn, and surfing a wave all require specific skills. As you've heard me say, how you move influences pain and injuries. But it also impacts your efficiency, speed, and power.

Good technique needs to be automatic. Cluttering your mind with the specifics of sports skills in a high-pressure situation is distracting and can bring about injury. Concentrating on how to shift your bicycle instead of the obstacles in the trail can easily send you down a steep slope. Your brain needs to be free of excess thoughts so you are ready to react. I often tell

training

my clients that during the race is not the time to be practicing technique; this should already be proficient. To gain this level of expertise, you must progress through the stages of "Motor Skill Acquisition," as developed by the psychology researchers Fitts and Posner (as cited in Ballou, 2011).[6] The three stages of Fitts and Posner's model are cognition, association, and autonomy.

Stage 1: Cognition

During the cognitive stage, you comprehend instructions and develop practice strategies. This is the time when the movement is broken down into component parts. When teaching classic style cross-country skiing, for instance, I'll start with body position, then move to balancing on the skis, leg movement, arm swing, and finally kick and glide. Each piece is practiced separately. Demonstrations of the techniques allow students to develop mental pictures to mimic. High mental effort is used during this phase of learning.

Stage 2: Association

During the associative stage, you begin to link movement components together. In this stage, I'll have my skiing students connect body position, balance, and glide. The associative phase is the time for more complex drills. Students refine their approach based on internal and external feedback of what produced the desired result—not falling and attaining glide—and what did not.

Stage 3: Autonomy

During the autonomous stage, your sports skills become more efficient and faster with less need for mental processing. At this point my students are skiing fluidly. This is the goal: automatic movement that does not require thought, allowing more energy and concentration for other tasks. Instead of focusing on the mechanics of a tennis serve, you can focus on where to put the ball on the opponent's side of the court.

Some of my worst gymnastics memories were of attending a competitive meet while still in the early associative phase of learning a new skill. Being nervous and having to think about how to do a trick while under the pressure of being judged is a recipe for disaster.

As you advance through these stages in developing your sports technique, the mental demand decreases. You are thinking less about how you move in each stage. Interestingly, in this model, there is little discussion of *feeling* the technique. As a coach, I find that most coaches talk too much. In my Professional Ski Instructor Association (PSIA) training, I was taught to say less and to keep my students skiing. Guided Discovery, a teaching style where you simply ask students to perform a skill without any verbal instruction, is one of my favorite ways to coach. Instead of filling my students' minds with words and ideas, I free them to experiment with different options and determine what brings the best result. This allows the skiers to tune in to their movements and discover how to perform most efficiently. I ask, "What did you do and feel when things went well?" And only afterward do we discuss the mechanics of the skills. Using this format for teaching, I can utilize the Motor Skill Acquisition stages without getting bogged down with overthinking and overanalyzing. Many times, *feeling* correct movement is the best feedback an instructor provides to her students.

This idea of feeling correct technique and allowing it to emerge naturally is central to the strategy of coaching that is advocated in the book *Inner Skiing.*[7] Authors Tim Gallwey and Dr. Robert Kriegel, pioneers in sports psychology, introduce the concepts of "Self 1"—the thinking brain, and "Self 2"—the *feeling* body with the innate ability to perform complex sports movements. They explain that frustration in learning a correct parallel turn in skiing, or any other sports technique, comes from the idea that you must acquire skills from somewhere outside yourself to succeed. They encourage us to believe in our skills and to stop limiting our potential through doubt. Does a bird doubt its ability to fly? Likewise, do you doubt your ability to swim, paddle, bike, climb, jump? All that you are learning when gaining a new sports skill through the stages of Motor Skill Acquisition—lies within you. To reach your full potential, you need to be able to quiet the commands of Self 1 ("Bend your knees! Relax your upper body! You can't make that turn!") and learn to trust Self 2. In the words of Gallwey and Kriegel,

training

Once we understand that it is the mind—Self 1—and its collection of self-concepts, doubts and fears accumulated over a lifetime which cause breakdowns and prevent optimal skiing, we can stop blaming our equipment, other people, snow conditions, and moguls. When Self 1 is in a quiet state, our awareness increases and we discover Self 2, that part of us that can respond to any situation instantaneously with its fullest capabilities.[7]

Regardless of how it is attained, good sports technique is important because it can determine whether you win or lose the race. I experienced this while competing in the *Valles Caldera Run*.

Nearing the top of the initial 1.5-mile climb was the aid station. I slowed to take a cup of Gatorade, and that's when she passed me. Oh crap! I had no idea another woman was so close! But I had to hydrate. The next section of the run consisted of steep ups and downs. I couldn't catch her. Every downhill I would gain some ground but just wasn't able to close the gap. Until . . . the long downhill. I didn't know the climbing was over, having never run the course before, but I saw the long stretch of downward-sloping road ahead. So, at the top, I leaned forward, relaxed, and let myself fly down. Thankfully, I was practiced in this technique. I soon passed her—as well as a couple of men—and I continued to pull away as I sped toward the finish line.

Sports technique is often overlooked in endurance training. Many athletes rationalize that their time is better spent developing their cardiovascular engines. Drills, which refine sports skills, are boring, and sometimes they don't seem important. It's much more fun to play your sport. However, it's not always the fittest athlete who wins the race. Rather, the skilled and practiced athlete sometimes takes home the top prize, even if that prize is just bragging rights between friends.

A few years ago I was in a classic cross-country ski race with a male friend. He had outstanding aerobic capacity, well above mine. Classic skiing has very precise technique. If your timing isn't right, you will repeatedly slip and become excruciatingly frustrated. Due to my countless hours of practicing classic drills and refining my technique, I skied well in the tricky race conditions, while my friend, more of a skate skier, struggled. As he flailed, I skied away.

Even if you are an advanced athlete, you can benefit from devoting time to refreshing and refining your skills. *Spending some of your precious training hours on technique is a good investment!* Sports technique is never truly mastered; it can always be improved. I regularly attend clinics to improve my personal sports skills. The off-season or early season is the best time for this practice.

To get the most out of your technique training, try using a video camera. Video feedback is one of the quickest ways to improve your technique. I often get dramatic results using this with clients who run and ski. I can explain the changes needed week after week, but once the student sees it, she rapidly makes the correction. Many of us are visual learners, which is why video is such a powerful tool. It just doesn't register when we hear it, but when we see it, we get it. After all, vision is our brain's dominant sense (Chapter 11).

Strategy 4: Counteract Sports Postures

Regardless of your sport, your body is repeatedly put into the same positions. Cyclists are hunched over and flex their spines, while dancers are continuously over-extending through their torsos. Runners and ball athletes also tend toward extension. If you want your body to continue to perform at an optimal level, these movements need to be counteracted. For an aligned body, cyclists need to extend their upper backs, while dancers, runners, and ball athletes need to flex their spines.

Consider your sport and what movements will best counter your frequently assumed positions. Your postural goal is a dynamic balance between the muscles on the front and the back of the body as well as left to right. Balanced muscles create a symmetrical skeleton and ideal joint alignment, which translates into more strength and power for the movements needed in your sport.

To counteract my cycling position and keep my body in balance, I thought doing yoga once a week was enough. *Nope!* Every time you play

training

sports, consider taking a few minutes as part of your cool down to move your body in the opposing direction. Golfers and tennis players are rotational athletes with a tendency to go one direction more than the other. After a round of golf or tennis match, put yourself into a position that twists you the other way. Following a run, get into a squat position with your chest touching your upper thighs. When you dismount the bike, stretch your upper spine in the reverse direction. Even just lying on the floor with your upper body supported will passively lengthen your spine and will relax your back and neck muscles, which have been held rigid while cycling. Finally, after nearly all sports, don't forget to stretch the front of your hips. Recall from Chapter 8 how tight hip flexors negatively impact pelvic position, hamstring length, and gluteal function.

Strategy 5: Embrace Cross-Training

Cross-training benefits your posture by counteracting your sports position, as described in Strategy 4. Your body grows stronger and more functionally balanced with diverse, tri-planar movement, as discussed in Chapter 12. Before I understood this concept, as a professional mountain biker, I trained by riding my bike all year round—to my detriment.

The year before I turned pro, I didn't even cross-country ski, which I love as much as mountain biking. My endurance racing started on Nordic skis. That year, I actually peddled my mountain bike up the snow-covered road to the ski area trails. I didn't venture out on my skinny skis at all. As it turned out, this was a poor decision for me physically, as you've read, and psychologically, because I didn't have any time off my bike. The result? I burned out, losing my ambition to race and ride later in the season, which my Sports Gremlin detested.

It's true that you need to practice your sport to gain fitness and proficiency, but maybe not to the point of excluding all else, all the time, including enjoyment during the off-season. In addition to the physical benefits, generating a little mental hunger for your sport can be a good thing. I'll even advise my clients to take a break from intensive sports training during the season to renew their desire for and dedication to training and competition.

Many athletes are stuck in the sagittal plane—moving the left and right sides of the body forward and backward, and straight ahead. This is the typical movement pattern of many sports and even walking. To reach peak performance, however, you need to be efficient in all three planes of motion. If your sport is dominant in the sagittal plane, you might consider cross-training by swimming breaststroke, which challenges function in the frontal plane, or inline skating, which incorporates rotational movement in the transverse plane. Maintain your ability to move your body efficiently in all three planes of motion on both your left and right sides to keep your body aligned, strong, and less likely to hurt or to become injured.

One of the best ways to regularly integrate these diverse, tri-planar movements into your training is through a functional conditioning program, as described in Chapter 12. While training hard at their sport, several of my athletic clients complement these efforts with functional strength workouts. Their exercises include movements and positions not typically assumed in their sport. I follow this advice myself, varying my training to give my body new postural messages and to engage different muscles with unfamiliar motions, which helps me to maintain structural symmetry.

Strategy 6: Honor Opponents

Competition stretches your abilities and tests your personal limits. When in pursuit of a victory, you'll put it all on the line to see how far you can go, how strong you are, and if you have what it takes to win. It is very hard to summon the same motivation and drive to expend your maximum effort on your own in a training session if your competitor is just a computer. My friend Thayla is a perfect example of this dichotomy.

Thayla transforms on the race start line. She jokes about her split personality: "Race day Thayla" and "Recreation Thayla." She thrives on racing, pushing herself harder and digging deeper than she ever could on her own. Having competitors brings out her best performance.

training

313

Competition isn't possible without opponents. What if you or your team were the only ones to show up for a match? Nearly all ball sports couldn't go on—basketball, baseball, football, tennis, racquetball, soccer, lacrosse, volleyball, rugby, etc. With nobody on the other side of the court or field, competition is impossible. Being the only individual contestant also greatly dampens your incentive. In races where I was the only woman, it just wasn't as much fun. I tended to hold back and avoid too much suffering, thinking, *I've already won the race anyway. Who am I competing against? I have no opponent!*

Early in my athletic career, I saw my rivals as threats. Since my hip injury, I've come to appreciate my opponents. I now realize that competition with others is an important part of my sporting events. Actually, I have a lot in common with my competitors. We share similar goals, priorities, and values. Instead of treating a challenger as a menace, someone needing to be squashed, I've expanded my view to see the person as an asset, someone who is motivating me to be a better athlete. Opponents are necessary. Competition with them is a positive aspect of the sporting experience. *Honor them!*[8]

Strategy 7: Relax!

Gripping the handlebars too tightly while mountain biking often causes you to overcorrect and crash. Tightening up when running can cause soreness and injury. Swinging harder at the golf ball nearly always creates a poor shot—and sometimes it leads to missing the ball completely. Letting go and taking it slower and easier is what is needed in these situations.

When things aren't going well, however, we tend to do the opposite: we work harder. We try to do more, which in many cases creates more tension in the system and makes things worse. Recall a time when you fell or made a mistake at an important event. What was your reaction? Like me, did you scramble and try to make up lost time by putting in even more effort, wasting tons of energy and not reaching your goal?

"We need to relax for maximum performance,"[8] says Jerry Lynch, Ph.D., sports psychologist and director of the TaoSports Center for Human Potential, and Warren Scott, M.D., family practice physician and founder of the Sports Medicine Division at Kaiser Permanente Medical Center in Santa Clara, CA. In their book *Running Within*, they go on to explain,

> Relaxed muscles are more fluid and contribute to greater coordination, strength and endurance. Relaxed bodies react more quickly. [...] Relaxed bodies burn less energy. [...] Relaxation lowers blood lactate. [...] Concentration and the ability to focus improve when you are relaxed, positively affecting your confidence.[8]

When I started to ride my mountain bike after my hip surgery, I still had pain in my back while climbing steep hills. The key to overcoming this was relaxation. When I felt my back muscles tightening and over working, I would breathe into my back. I'd visualize the muscles stretching and releasing. The discomfort would then subside.

Relaxation is also needed mentally and emotionally. When my back would tighten, my mind would stiffen, too. Panic, doubt, and fear would fill my brain. Just like the physical muscle tightness, I had to relax my mind and release these negative thoughts.

You've come a long way to this point in your journey! Your pain and injury are managed, and you have learned appropriate sports training strategies to keep you healthy for the long-term. The only thing left is to get back out there and play again. That's the final topic covered in the last chapter.

training

Summary

This chapter provided seven strategies for your sports performance.

Strategy 1: Have a Flexible Plan

Try to avoid being a slave to your daily workout log. Reap greater gains in your training by listening to your body and coordinating your hardest efforts with the days you have the greatest energy and motivation.

Strategy 2: Balance Stress and Recovery

Fitness is only gained when the body is given appropriate rest; strive to let go of the idea that you always need to be doing and pushing in order to advance.

Strategy 3: Refine Sports Technique

Efficiency in your movements is gained through repetition of correct patterns where you tune in, feel, and trust your body's innate ability to perform complicated sports skills.

Strategy 4: Counteract Sports Postures

Practicing the same sport over and over creates a specific pattern of strain on your body that needs to be neutralized through the practice of consistent opposing movements to prevent unwanted postural adaptations, pain, performance declines and greater injury risk.

Strategy 5: Embrace Cross-Training

Integrating different tri-planar activities into your training benefits your body physically. It also develops mental hunger and motivation for your primary sport to avoid burnout.

Strategy 6: Honor Opponents

For the game to go on, you need someone to compete against; opponents bring out your best effort and should be appreciated for the necessary role they play in sports.

Strategy 7: Relax!
Being free of physical, mental, and emotional tension and anxiety leads to your best sports performance. *Stay calm to excel!*

These strategies are based on respect for yourself while simultaneously improving your athletics.

training

Game Winning Strategies

1. Evaluate Your Sports Performance Strategies

Listed below are journal questions for each strategy. You may find you are doing great in some areas but have room for improvement in others. Feel free to skip questions that don't apply to you. For the questions where you find work is needed, also write the first simple step you can take toward success.

Strategy 1: Have a Flexible Plan
How flexible is your training plan?
What are the characteristics of your Sports Gremlin?

Describe your Sports Gremlin in detail—the gender, appearance, words and tone used, as many details as possible. Just bringing awareness to your Sports Gremlin can be the first step in releasing his or her hold over you.

Strategy 2: Balance Stress and Recovery
How well are you balancing your stress and recovery?
What recovery rituals do you have—or want to put in place—for each of your energy capacities: physical, emotional, mental, and spiritual?

Strategy 3: Refine Sports Technique
Are all your sports techniques automatic and refined?
If not, how are you going to reach this level of achievement with these skills?
What impact would improved body mechanics and form have on your sports performance?

Strategy 4: Counteract Sports Postures
What are the positions and motions you frequently perform in your sport?
How are you counteracting your sports postures?

Strategy 5: Embrace Cross-Training
How are you incorporating cross-training into your training program?
What planes of motion—sagittal, frontal, transverse—are you including in your cross-training?

Strategy 6: Honor Opponents
How do you view your opponents?
What would it take to see your opponents as a greater asset to your performance?

Strategy 7: Relax!
When performing, how easy is it for you to stay relaxed?
What athletic situations trigger anxiety and panic?
How might you improve your ability to let go during competition?

2. <u>Define Your Own Strategies</u>

In this chapter I shared with you the wholistic strategies I found important for sports performance, but there is always room for more and different options.

Reflecting on what you have read, combined with your previous experiences and understanding, what additional strategies would you add to what I have provided?

3. <u>Review Your Strategy Rating</u>

Now that you have read the additional strategies for wholistic sports training and added some of your own, take a look back at Chapter 13 and consider the number you assigned to the strategy slice of the Wheel of Sports Performance.

With the additional knowledge you have gained, do you agree with the rating you initially made, or should it be changed?

training

15

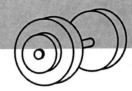

Emerging as a New Athlete

*Y*our pain and injury have changed you. In a very obvious way, your body is physically different. But your mind has also been altered. You no longer think or act the same way. Hopefully, after reading this book, your long-held beliefs about your body, healing, and sports have been challenged. To recover, you have had to modify expectations, rearrange priorities, set new goals, adopt a different perspective, and consider alternative approaches to healing and training.

The choices you make from here going forward will direct your path. It is up to you now. Behave as you did before your injury and possibly end up hurt again, or use the knowledge and tools you have gained in the previous pages to reach another destination. From now on, you are the author writing the story. Use your story to create a reality that will take you where you ultimately want to go, as I discussed in Chapter 1. Will you re-enter the sports world transformed and reach greater heights than before? *I hope so. I did, and I know you can, too!*

Conquering Your Fear of Re-injury

As you resume sports, your primary fear is most likely re-injury. You may have been through extensive rehabilitation, unable to play your sport, and you don't want to go back to that place again any time soon. Unfortunately, this fear increases your stress, which raises your risk of re-injury, according to research by Jean Williams Ph.D., Emeritus Professor of Psychology at the University of Arizona. Williams found that high stress and many daily hassles make you more prone to injury. Her research showed that athletes under stress find it hard to focus and maintain attention. In addition, she observed these athletes held increased muscle tension throughout their bodies.[1] As you read in Chapter 14, relaxed muscles elevate performance and lower injury risk.

Further, a study by Podlog and Eklund found fear of re-injury to be higher for athletes with recurring injuries than athletes with one-time injuries. Their research also showed that injured athletes returning to sport were stressed by several factors, including "(1) increased intensity of competition, (2) injury flare-ups/injury to another part of the body, (3) not making/getting dropped from teams and (4) reduced confidence."[2]

So, here again, is a link between stress, sports, and healing. I can't overemphasize how important it is to keep your stress in check for so many reasons. Hopefully, you developed some good stress-relieving rituals—like journaling, deep breathing, meditation, reading, socializing—throughout your healing process and are implementing them regularly.

In addition to the fears I've already listed, which are all normal and common, you may also be afraid of not being as good as you were before injury. Your mind may still view yourself as the athlete you were prior to being hurt. You don't want to embarrass yourself and have your peers see your weakness. And, you want to live up to that image for yourself and those around you. As I shared in Chapter 2, I had this fear, and I didn't want to ride with anyone who might criticize me for my lack of fitness.

Here's the truth. Although you might still be defining and judging yourself by these criteria, your true friends and family don't hinge your value as a person on your athletics. More than likely, you will receive overwhelming support for being back out on the field. If you don't, you might want to reconsider your affiliations. Many times, the negative perceptions you *think* you notice coming from others are merely projections of your mind with no substance to back them up.

After being off my bike for over a year, I knew it was going to be hard to go back. I shared all the fears and doubts you likely do. Surprisingly, it was easier than I expected. The joy of being back on the bike and feeling healthy again far outweighed my hesitations. Due to the rehab I had done, I was stronger in new ways. My fitness gradually came back, and if I wanted to, I could focus on training again. In the beginning, though, just being able to enjoy riding without pain was a thrill that I wanted to relish for a while.

When your fear of re-injury is conquered, your athletic confidence grows. Confidence in your body comes from knowing it is aligned and strong with optimal muscle biomechanics. This confidence is built through respecting and tuning in to your sensations. Your ability to connect with and listen to your body allows you to take appropriate preventive actions and head off any early signs of injury. Knowing your pain, not reacting with instant panic, helps you make smart choices and keeps your body safe from harm. Confidence in your sport is gained over time through gradual progression, good technique, adequate recovery and consistent small successes.

Learning Athletic Toughness

Throughout my years as a competitive athlete, I thought I was tough by pushing through the pain. This is not athletic toughness, though many still hold this belief.

As an example, while competing in a multi-day mountain bike stage race, a rider crashed and suffered a rotator cuff (shoulder) injury during one of the first few days in the race. Although she was only able to ride holding the handle bars with one hand, she vowed to finish the race, despite her pain and injury. The impressed race announcer told her story to all the racers, holding her up as an example for others to follow. Despite her determination, the injured rider wasn't able to finish the race, as her riding was too slow to make the time cuts—a blessing in disguise for her body.

For many athletes it is harder *not* to compete when injured. Previously, I was not tough enough to sit by and watch others participate. I made bad choices, pushing my body when it needed recovery. The drive to be in the action is so strong that our minds can create elaborately skewed logic that convinces us it is okay to go out and play when we hurt.

The tough athlete is not the one who can endure the most pain! Rather, my definition of athletic toughness is having the integrity to listen to your body, make self-respecting choices, and think beyond today's event. Instead of being tough, I often took the easy, though self-destructive, path. My career-ending hip injury taught me athletic toughness.

training

323

Three years after my hip surgery, in July 2011, I was registered for the single-speed cross-country National Off Road Bike Association (NORBA) Nationals. I had a bad fall in my pre-ride the day before the race. I lost my balance on a narrow uphill section and tumbled down the side of the mountain—sliding about 50 feet below the trail on my back. I had numerous cuts and bruises, but the worst was my lower back, my site of chronic pain, which went into an excruciating spasm.

To race, or not, was the critical decision that I had to make— quickly. The pre-injury Jessica would have stepped up to the starting line without hesitation. However, I was different now, so I didn't know what to do. Here's the debate I had with myself that day:

Should I race? This is the question that needs an answer TODAY. Despite my pain and incapacity, I have paid $120 to participate. On top of that, I renewed my NORBA license ($70) for the first time in five years to have this opportunity. I have dedicated myself to train for the event. And this was to be the start of my comeback. I'm already here at my home in Hailey, ID, only 10 miles from the venue, evacuated from my permanent residence in Los Alamos, NM, due to wildfire. It will be fun and will give me a gauge of my fitness. I have never raced with more than a couple of women in my field, and the best in the country will be at the event.

Then again, maybe I shouldn't. It will be very painful. I'm not able to lift my leg over my bike saddle without wincing, and I haven't even been able to get into position to pedal. Yes, mountain bike racing is supposed to hurt, but to this degree? My riding will be tentative. I will be overly cautious on the course, feeling my fresh wounds and not wanting to take another fall on them. I could exacerbate my hip injury that I have diligently worked to repair for the last four years. Right lower back pain is what brought my career to a halt several years ago.

I know my hips and pelvis are out of alignment due to the crash. Is it really a good idea to repeatedly push one challenging gear around a course with over 2500 ft of climbing in this crooked position? Each powerful revolution of the pedals will be reinforcing my misalignments and compensations. Riding single-speed, I'll have to dismount and remount my bike many times, which is currently a very difficult and painful maneuver. And, I'll be standing on the pedals, pushing and pulling with every aching muscle in my body just to keep the wheels turning.

But I really don't want a "Did Not Start" (DNS) next to my name on the results. I've told people I'm racing. I'd feel like I was letting them down and don't want to explain why I didn't participate. It's such a hard decision. The battle rages between emotions and logic . . .

In the end, I was tough: I didn't race. And my Sports Gremlin was furious. But I wasn't letting him dictate my behavior anymore. He could throw a tantrum all he wanted, and I'd just stand by and watch his shenanigans. I realized that I had made up my Sports Gremlin. He was not me, but a creation of my mind. He was a fantasy that I could choose to listen to or not. By distancing myself from him and just observing his actions without buying into his harmful rhetoric, I could make peace with my Sports Gremlin.

That day, I made a decision I have stuck with ever since. A race is not worth it if it jeopardizes my body. It took four joint surgeries and years of healing for me to come to this realization. *Why would I want to risk more pain, endure more rehab and take more time off my bike and enjoyment of other sports, just for one race?* It doesn't make any sense. All the rationalizing in the world about money spent, people disappointed, training wasted (and on and on) will not make it okay. You are the one who is most upset and frustrated. Every time you make a smart decision that nurtures yourself, you are displaying athletic toughness, and you are building your confidence.

Finding the Opportunity in Your Injury

Initially, I was at a loss with my hip and back pain. My life had been turned upside down. I didn't know what to make of my situation or how to move forward. I needed help and a new perspective. So, I started reading. I picked up one of the recommended books from my wellness coaching program, *Man's Search for Meaning* by Dr. Viktor E. Frankl, M.D., Ph.D., Austrian neurologist and psychiatrist, founder of Logotherapy, and Holocaust survivor. *Wow!* I highly recommend reading this book. It was life-changing for me. The book tells the inspiring story of Frankl's years

training

in Nazi concentration camps, where he continued to see beauty and feel optimistic despite the dismal conditions and ever-present threat of death.[3] His book is sure to help you realize the good in your life and increase your gratitude and appreciation for what you have.

Frankl's book started to shift my perceptions about my circumstances. I had so much to be thankful for, yet I was choosing to focus my attention on my pain and loss. It took many more books, most of which have been mentioned throughout this book, on positive psychology, fear, motivation, success, happiness, meditation, stress, transitions, and others, to move me from an attitude of *woe is me, my life is over,* to realizing there might actually be an opportunity in this experience.

Remember the Whole Life Grid from Chapter 3 or the Wheel of Life from Chapter 13? I needed to be reminded that there was a lot more to me and who I was than just my sports. Many aspects of my life had been shut down because I didn't have time for them while pursuing competitive athletics. I needed to reignite these areas.

After my injuries, while healing, I explored many new and rewarding activities, one of which was attending a show at the Santa Fe Opera with friends after years of driving by the Opera House and thinking, *I really should check that out sometime.* This experience raised my appreciation for the arts and inspired me to include more of these activities—symphony performances, live plays, art exhibits—in my life, even after my injury. While laid up, I also took guitar lessons for the second time, started meditating, and experimented in the kitchen with several new recipes. Additionally, I tended the garden and finished several projects around the house with my husband. Following my recovery, I didn't stick with all these activities—guitar just doesn't seem to be for me—but the garden expands each year, and Ken and I persist in making new meals from our crops.

The biggest opportunity in my injury, however, was regarding my career. Frankl's theory—Logotherapy—is based on the premise that we are ultimately driven to find meaning in life: "According to logotherapy, this striving to find a meaning in one's life is the primary motivational force in man."[3] My injury gave me meaning and direction for my work.

I had never loved the attention of being a professional athlete. In some ways, I felt I was selfish to spend so much time for myself riding a bike. I persisted because I truly enjoyed the sport. Also, my motivation to gain significance through mountain biking and identify as an athlete was strong.

I didn't know what I'd do without that. Training and racing had become my way of life. My social circle consisted mainly of my teammates and fellow cyclists. I didn't know what else to do; I didn't know another way to live. I'd ask myself, *What am I contributing to society by riding my bike?* Some inspiration, I supposed, but it felt hollow to me. I wanted to give more. My chronic pain showed me how.

While injured, without the distraction of cycling, I had to face the reality of being at a job I disliked, one that gave me no satisfaction. After months of debating, and with looming doubts, I made a hard decision with the encouragement and support of my dear husband. I quit my secure, government job to pursue my own business full time and work in a field I am passionate about. Although scary at the time, this choice has been one of the best decisions I have ever made in my life. I am now working in harmony with my deepest values. I am using my athletic experience and my continually expanding knowledge about the body, healing, and sports to help others. Importantly, I'm more motivated to continue riding my bike, and I enjoy sharing my love of mountain biking with others through teaching. I want to be a role model. I want people to see that they can overcome their chronic pain and injury to pursue their dreams.

I know it might be hard to view your injury as an opportunity, but there might be a positive side, something to be learned that will benefit you. Upon reflection of his recovery, my client Vic, who had paralyzing pain in his low back and was diagnosed with three herniated discs, arthritis, stenosis, and sciatica, was grateful for his pain. Here is what he had to say:

After four months of slow but continuous progress through daily work, I am actually thankful for the experience [of paralyzing back pain] and looking forward to a new life with a strong body, free of the accumulation of pain from 60 years of intense athletic spurts interrupted by long periods of sitting incorrectly at a desk. In other words, I am thankful for the most painful month I've ever experienced because it slapped me in the face with the news that sooner or later, one needs to care for the body, and sooner is better. In addition to pain-free movement, my exercise regimen has me now gratefully returning to riding my mountain bike, skiing, and golf. My therapy has caused me to slow down and train for perfection and not for

training

adrenaline. Maybe best of all, my now aspirin-free golf game seems to have lost a few strokes, a miracle I can only attribute to a better aligned body yielding better results.

Other clients have also found opportunity and meaning in their injury. One injured client began coaching her daughter's diving team. This deepened their relationship and fulfilled my client's need to be in a sports environment. Another injured client began marriage counseling to strengthen the bond with his spouse; he turned a marriage heading for divorce into a joyful union.

You can also use your extra time to continue to progress in your sport. There is more to being a great athlete than hard workouts. Are you knowledgeable about your equipment? How about your sports technique? Do you need to update your training plan? The mental practice of visualization has been shown to aid performance while injured. Olympic diver Laura Wilkinson benefitted from visualization before the *2000 Summer Olympic Games* while healing from a severe foot injury. Since she couldn't dive, she trained by using mental images of her dives. Despite not being able to physically do the movements for a couple months, through visualization, she was able to train such precise technique that she earned the gold medal in the platform competition.[4]

Growing From Your Pain

You grow stronger when overcoming your greatest challenges. Having this difficulty is part of your learning process in life. You do not grow as a person in your comfort zone when all is going smoothly. It is in the rough patches of life where you expand. We need to embrace these experiences for what they are and float with them. Not fight, not try to fix, just release and allow things to happen.

How have you grown and what have you learned while being injured? My client Maurine told me she has learned to be calmer and more patient. She no longer pushes through what she cannot control. Her pain is inconsistent and unpredictable, so she listens to her body carefully, accepts her circumstances, and just relaxes and goes with the flow. Lynn connected with her body and discovered how to see the gray shades of her pain. She learned that even though she still had pain some days, she could manage it, and that she preferred to live with it rather than run from it. Bernice gained body awareness and learned how to relax her muscles to stop the discomfort in her back. Tarik realized he needed to keep his hips mobile to reduce his lower back and knee pain. Trish attained balance by connecting with her spiritual and emotional sides. She also began respecting her body and stopped pushing through her pain. Helen developed appreciation for the underlying cause of her back pain, the postural asymmetries in her spine. Although the surgery took away her immediate pain, she committed to changing her alignment to prevent another episode. After years of treating her symptom, Marilyn found relief from her plantar fasciitis by treating her whole body as an integrated unit. Jaqueline learned there is more to life than running. She tried new sports—mountain biking, cross-country skiing, hiking—which brought her satisfaction, enjoyment, and lasting friendships. Sandra gained confidence in her body and wasn't afraid to dream about future athletic adventures again.

One of my biggest lessons was learning to slow down and pace myself, both in sports and life. Many of us burn ourselves out because we do not know how to pace. We frantically jump from one thing to the next with no break. Just like in Aesop's Fable, *The Tortoise and the Hare,*[5] slow and steady wins the race. Sprinting, then walking, is not as effective as a moderate, consistent pace. While running a trail marathon, I experienced this first hand: I kept a consistent pace and repeatedly passed—and eventually left behind—athletes who were inconsistent in their pace.

Through my holistic healing journey, I learned to stop doing and to "just be" for the first time in my life. I realized that I kept myself distracted—and my sympathetic nervous system (SNS) fully charged—through sports training, work, and endless tasks because I was afraid to be still and know myself. I thought I was happy and content when I was always on the go. But my chronic pain forced my stillness. It allowed me to experience myself fully and discover another way of being in the world with a calm, relaxed, and positive presence.

If you believe things happen for a reason, then this injury has a purpose for you. It may be a simple lesson, or it may mark a life-changing event. It should not just make you miserable. Let it help you grow in your life. The growth may be around your sport, but it is likely broader than that.

training

Staying Pain and Injury Free

Taking care of your body and practicing the skills you have learned in this book shouldn't stop when the pain goes away. Staying pain and injury free requires a lifestyle change. From now on I hope you'll view pain as a helpful warning; tune in and listen closely to your body; maintain alignment—physically, mentally, emotionally, and spiritually; sense your environment; develop your core; build functional strength; train wholistically; and breathe deeply from your diaphragm. These techniques have worked for me and many of my clients. They should work for you, too.

You can do more than you think you can! I recall this sentiment being expressed during the *Leadville 100* mountain bike pre-race briefing. Refuse to confine yourself with conventional beliefs. It's not too late, and you're not too old. Don't accept physical limitations or agree that aging brings inevitable pain and immobility. Many people will blame injuries and pain on their age. I'm here to tell you that giving up sports is not a certainty of growing older. Sports are not to blame for your injuries, either. Your body is designed to move and play throughout your lifetime. As I've described throughout this book, it is the *position and condition* of the body brought into sports that matters and predicts an athlete's performance and injury risk, *not* the sports you play, and *not* your age. The longer you have been playing, and the more injuries you have accrued, the more out of balance your body tends to become. Advancing years, then, increase the chances of your body being asymmetrical, but that can be improved, as you've read. And when you improve your alignment, you can reach new athletic heights.

My Athletic Story Continues

As I said in the beginning, all I wanted was to keep up with my husband, Ken, while mountain biking. That hasn't changed. I still love riding with him, though it often continues to feel like I'm just constantly chasing his back wheel. So, I found a solution: a two-person multi-day mountain bike stage race where you are penalized an hour in your race time if you are separated from your partner by more than two minutes on the course. *Now, Ken had to ride with me!* And, even better, he had incentive to assist me to keep us together and better our time.

In 2016, a decade after my career ending hip injury, Ken and I entered the *joBerg2c*, www.joberg2c.co.za, a nine day, 500-mile mountain bike race from Johannesburg, South Africa to the coast of the Indian Ocean. We chose this event because we had always wanted to do one of these races, the dates corresponded with our 20th wedding anniversary, the terrain didn't look too difficult, and it was in a very cool location. I was nervous about signing up for such a big event, which required extensive travel and necessitated that I perform jointly with my husband. I had doubts about my body: *What if I had pain and couldn't sustain the repeated efforts?* It was going to be tough: nine consecutive days of riding; 50+ miles at each stage; multiple demanding climbs, floating bridges, and wild animals. I'd never done anything like this before. But after all the work I had done to heal, and after all the specific training I had done for the event, I felt strong and ready for the ride. I decided that regardless of our results in South Africa, I had won, just because I had gotten to this point.

As it turned out, my body showed excellent resilience and met each daily challenge. We did struggle the first few days, still jet lagged and adjusting to the local cuisine. At the end of day three, we seriously questioned our decision to enter this event, as we both realized this was the hardest athletic endeavor either of us had ever undertaken. Things improved on stage 4 as the race course changed from the long, grinding district roads and headed into the mountains and more technical single-track riding. We found our groove. We were getting stronger and feeling better every day. Ken was feeling so good that on stage 6 he started giving me assistance. A strategy used by the teams is for the faster rider to push the slower rider, or for the slower rider to hang on to the faster rider's back pocket. After riding hard and helping Ken on the earlier stages, I wasn't sure about being pushed. I

training

331

saw it as a sign of weakness, but I couldn't deny that I appreciated the help. We never could have gone as quickly without using this tactic.

To overcome my feelings of resentment and inadequacy about being pushed, I recalled one of the healing lessons my beloved dog, Coral, had taught me: "It's okay to accept help from others—swallow your ego and be vulnerable." This memory changed my perspective from being insulted to being grateful for Ken's strength and helping hand. Just that little boost from him allowed me to keep spinning my gears and powering up the climbs. In addition to giving me physical encouragement, his nudge lifted me mentally, emotionally, and spiritually.

As the days passed, we were slowly moving up in our stage finishes. Upon realizing we placed 11th in the mixed pairs category on stage 7, I set my sights on breaking into the top 10. We didn't have a shot at a good overall result with our poor performance on the first few days, but a top 10 stage finish was within our reach. Although we gave it our best effort on stage 8, which I thought was well suited to our strengths with lots of technical climbing, we were 11th again. With only one mostly downhill stage to go, I didn't have much hope that we'd achieve our goal. Thankfully, my ever-optimistic husband was by my side and was determined to get us into the top 10. His positive attitude was infectious: it turned my pessimism around. After a very hard ride on that last day with rain, strong winds, and crossing the longest and scariest floating bridge to the finish—*we did it! We were 10th!*

In my mind, completing the *joBerg2c* marked the end of my healing journey. There is still more recovery work to be done—I always want to keep improving—but the bigger issues, the ones that had been limiting my sports, are now controlled. I continue to use the tools I described in this book, and I can now progress to spending more of my time on the strength building and training regiments instead of only rehab exercises, though these are still a large and important part of my daily program. I have gone from pain and disability back to competition and having fun on my bike again. It is a great feeling.

Time to start the next chapter in my athletic life . . .

Summary

You are a different athlete following an injury. You have grown better and stronger—physically, mentally, emotionally, and spiritually. It is natural to be afraid of re-injury when returning to sports. With all you have learned and all the work you have done, you can be confident that you are prepared to engage safely in sport again. Playing through the pain is not tough. Rather, athletic toughness is being strong enough not to push when you're hurting. Playing in pain will only lead to poor outcomes, like more time in rehab and days on the sidelines. Injuries can provide opportunities for other activities, new priorities, or needed changes in your life direction. Personal growth happens during the challenging times of your life. You want to emerge stronger following these circumstances. Allow yourself to expand and grow from this experience. Once you go back to sports, don't forget all the lessons you have learned in these pages. Staying pain and injury free requires lifelong diligence.

Be empowered to take charge of your health and future through the choices you make today about your body, healing, and training. Choose well so you can have a long life filled with energy, joy, vitality, youthfulness, and strength. Pedal on to your dream destination.

Best Wishes, and Good Luck!

training

Game Winning Strategies

1. Reflect on Your Progress

Here is a final set of journal questions to help you capture the transformation you have made through your healing journey. You can imagine how you would have answered these questions before reading this book compared with your current responses.

What is the opportunity or meaning in your injury and pain?

What have you learned and how have you grown through your injury experience?

Which of the strategies that you learned in this book are you going to implement and stick with for the long-term to keep yourself pain and injury free so you can stay in the game for life?

What are you grateful for about your injury and healing journey?

2. Join The Pain Free Athlete Community

Sign-up for The Pain Free Athlete Newsletter: www.thepfathlete.com

Write a book review on The Pain Free Athlete Facebook Page: www.facebook.com/painfreeathlete

Subscribe to The Pain Free Athlete YouTube Channel: www.youtube.com/user/ThePainFreeAthlete

Follow The Pain Free Athlete on Twitter: www.twitter.com/painfreeathlete

Connect with Jessica on LinkedIn: www.linkedin.com/in/jessicakisiel

Write Jessica an Email: jessica@thepfathlete.com

training

Endnotes

Introduction

1. Cook, G. (2003). *Athletic body in balance: Optimal movement skills and conditioning for performance.* Champaign, IL: Human Kinetics.

2. Bowman, K. (2014). *Move your DNA: Restore health through natural movement.* Carlsborg, WA: Propriometrics Press.

3. Postural Restoration Institute® (PRI). (2016). *Impingement & instability course.* Lincoln, NE: Postural Restoration Institute® (PRI).

4. Benson, H. (1975). *The relaxation response.* New York, NY: HarperTorch™.

5. Rankin, L. (2014). *Mind over medicine: Scientific proof that you can heal yourself.* Carlsbad, CA: Hay House, Inc.

6. Sisgold, S. (2015). *Whole body intelligence: Get out of your head and into your body to achieve greater wisdom, confidence, and success.* New York, NY: Rodale Books.

7. Loehr, J. & Schwartz, T. (2001). The making of a corporate athlete. *Harvard Business Review, 176*, 120-128.

Chapter 1

1. Postural Restoration Institute® (PRI). (2015). *PRI integration for fitness and movement course: Restoring tri-planar performance through respiration and alternating reciprocal activity.* Lincoln, NE: Postural Restoration Institute® (PRI).

2. The Egoscue Method®, www.egoscue.com, 12230 El Camino Real #110, San Diego, CA 92130, (800) 995-8434.

3. Egoscue, P. (1998). *Pain free: A revolutionary method for stopping chronic pain.* New York, NY: Bantam Books.

4. Postural Restoration Institute® (PRI), www.posturalrestoration.com, 5255 R Street, Lincoln, NE 68504, (402) 467-4111.

5. Loher, J. (2007). *The power of story: Change your story, change your destiny in business and in life.* New York, NY: Free Press.

Chapter 2

1. Moseley, G. L. (2012). *Painful yarns: Metaphors & stories to help understand the biology of pain.* Minneapolis, MN: OPTP.

2. Kabat-Zinn, J. (1990). *Full catastrophe living: Using the wisdom of your body and mind to face stress, pain, and illness.* New York, NY: Dell Publishing.

3. TED. (2011, Nov. 21). *Lorimer Moseley - Why things hurt* [Video file]. Retrieved from www.youtube.com/watch?v=gwd-wLdIHjs

4. Sarno, J. E. (1991). *Healing back pain: The mind-body connection.* New York, NY: Grand Central Publishing.

5. Moseley, G. L. (2013). *Explain pain* (2nd ed.). Adelaide City West, South Australia: Noigroup Publications.

6. Jensen, M. C., Brant-Zawadzki, M. N., Obuchowski, N., Modic, M. T., Malkasian, D., & Ross, J. S. (1994). Magnetic resonance imaging of the lumbar spine in people without back pain. *New England Journal of Medicine, 331,* 69-73.

7. Bianco, T., Malo, S. & Orlick, T. (1999). Sports injury and illness: Elite skiers describe their experiences. *Research Quarterly for Exercise and Sport, 70,* 157-169.

8. Louw, A. (2013). *Why do I hurt?: A patient book about the neuroscience of pain.* Story City, IA: International Spine and Pain Institute.

Chapter 3

1. Kübler-Ross, E. (1997). *On death and dying.* New York, NY: Scribner. (Original work published in 1969).

2. Brewer, B. W. (1994). Review and critique of models of psychological adjustment to athletic injury. *Journal of Applied Sports Psychology, 6*(1), 87-100.

3. Hanin, Y. L. (Ed.). (2000). *Emotions in sport.* Champaign, IL: Human Kinetics.

4. TED. (2007, Jan. 16). *Why we do what we do | Tony Robbins* [Video file]. Retrieved from www.youtube.com/watch?v=Cpc-t-Uwv1I

5. McLeod, S. A. (2016). Maslow's hierarchy of needs. *Simple Psychology.* Retrieved from www.simplypsychology.org/maslow.html

6. Cherry, K. (2016, June 19). Biography of Abraham Maslow (1908-1970). Retrieved from www.verywell.com/ biography-of-abraham-maslow-1908-1970-2795524

7. Jeffers, S. (2006). *Feel the fear . . . and do it anyway: Dynamic techniques for turning fear, indecision, and anger into power, action, and love.* New York, NY: Ballantine Books.

8. Marano, H. E. (2003, June 20). Our brain's negativity bias: Why our brains are more highly attuned to negative news. *Psychology Today.* Retrieved from www.psychologytoday.com/articles/200306/our-brains-negative-bias

9. Sapolsky, R. M. (2004). *Why zebras don't get ulcers: The acclaimed guide to stress, stress-related diseases, and coping.* New York, NY: Holt Paperbacks.

10. Peterson, C. & Seligman, M. (1984). Causal explanations as a risk factor for depression: Theory and evidence. *Psychological Review, 91,* 347-74.

11. Seligman, M. E. P. (2002). *Authentic happiness: Using the new positive psychology to realize your potential for lasting fulfillment.* New York, NY: Free Press.

12. Seligman, M. E. P. (2006). *Learned optimism: How to change your mind and your life.* New York, NY: Vintage Books.

13. Ievleva, L. & Orlick, T. (1991). Mental links to enhanced healing: An exploratory study. *The Sports Psychologist, 5,* 25-40.

14. Pargman, D. (Ed.). (2007). *Psychological bases of sports injuries.* Morgantown, WV: West Virginia University.

15. Ford, I. W., Gordon, S., & Eklund, R. C. (2000). An examination of psychosocial variables moderating the relationship between life stress and injury time-loss among athletes of a high standard. *Journal of Sports Sciences, 18*(5), 301-312. www.tandfonline.com/doi/abs/10.1080/026404100402368

16. Grove, J. R., Stewart, R. M. L., & Gordon, S. (1990, October). Emotional reactions of athletes to knee rehabilitation. Paper presented at the annual meeting of the Australian Sports Medicine Federation, Alice Springs.

17. Lyubomirsky, S., Sheldon, K. M., & Schkade, D. (2005). Pursuing happiness: The architecture of sustainable change. *Review of General Psychology, 9,* 111-131.

18. Thomas, P. & Shea, A. (2005). *Petria Thomas: Swimming against the tide.* Available from www.audible.com/pd/ Bios-Memoirs/Petria-Thomas-Audiobook/B002V1NMQA/ ref=a_search_c4_1_1_srTtl?qid=1460394895&sr=1-1

19. Wellcoaches® Corporation. (2006). Lesson 5: Wellness planning. Wellness Coach® Training Manual. Wellesley, MA: Wellcoaches® Corporation.

20. Wellcoaches® Corporation. (2005). Wellness vision coaching tool. Wellness Coach® Training Manual. Wellesley, MA: Wellcoaches® Corporation.

Chapter 4

1. Byrne, R. (2010). *The power (The secret).* New York, NY: Atria Books.

2. Rankin, L. (2014). *Mind over medicine: Scientific proof that you can heal yourself.* Carlsbad, CA: Hay House, Inc.

3. The Egoscue Method®, www.egoscue.com, 12230 El Camino Real #110, San Diego, CA 92130, (800) 995-8434.

4. Egoscue, P. (1998). *Pain free: A revolutionary method for stopping chronic pain.* New York, NY: Bantam Books.

5. Coren, S. (2013, Mar. 14). Which emotions do dogs actually experience?: Dogs have the same emotions as a human 2 year-old child. *Psychology Today.* Retrieved from www.psychologytoday.com/blog/canine-corner/201303/which-emotions-do-dogs-actually-experience

6. Fredrickson, B. L. (2009). *Positivity: Top notch research reveals the upward spiral that will change your life.* New York, NY: Three Rivers Press.

7. Laughlin, T. (2004). *Total immersion: The revolutionary way to swim better, faster, and easier.* New York, NY: Fireside.

Chapter 5

1. Egoscue, P. (1998). *Pain free: A revolutionary method for stopping chronic pain.* New York, NY: Bantam Books.

2. Jensen, K. (n.d.). Musculoskeletal system. Retrieved from www.biologyreference.com/Mo-Nu/Musculoskeletal-System.html

3. Myers, T. W. (2014). *Anatomy Trains®: Myofascial meridians for manual & movement therapists.* New York, NY: Churchill Livingston.

4. Gunther Von Hagens' Body Worlds: The original exhibition of real human bodies. (n.d.). Mission of the exhibitions. Retrieved from www.bodyworlds.com/en/exhibitions/mission_exhibitions.html

5. Myers, T. W. (2012). *Fascia and the Anatomy Trains webinar series* [Webinar]. Retrieved from www.anatomytrains.com/product/fascia-and-the-anatomy-trains-webinar-videos

6. Myers, T. (2012, Dec. 4). *What is tensegrity - Tom Myers* [Video file]. Retrieved from www.youtube.com/watch?v=BzgxYpDyO0M

7. James Weldon Johnson. Dem bones. Bascomb Lunsford. 1928.

8. Comana, F. (2011). *ACE's functional training and assessment workshop.* San Diego, CA: American Council on Exercise.

9. Kendall, F., McCreary, E., Provance, P., Rodgers, M. & Romani, W. (2005). *Muscles: Testing and function with posture and pain* (5th ed.). Baltimore, MD: Lippincott Williams & Wilkins.

Chapter 6

1. The Egoscue Method®, www.egoscue.com, 12230 El Camino Real #110, San Diego, CA 92130, (800) 995-8434.

2. Egoscue, P. (2001). *The Egoscue Method of health through motion: A revolutionary program that lets you rediscover the body's power to protect and rejuvenate itself.* New York, NY: Quill.

3. Wirhed, R. (2006). *Athletic ability and the anatomy of motion* (3rd ed.). New York, NY: Mosby.

4. Egoscue University®. (2007). EM 201 Posture identification course. San Diego, CA: Egoscue University®.

5. Kendall, F., McCreary, E., Provance, P., Rodgers, M. & Romani, W. (2005). *Muscles: Testing and function with posture and pain* (5th ed.). Baltimore, MD: Lippincott Williams & Wilkins.

6. Postural Restoration Institute® (PRI). (2014). *Myokinematic restoration course: An integrated approach to treatment of patterned lumbo-pelvic-femoral pathomechanics.* Lincoln, NE: Postural Restoration Institute® (PRI).

7. Bowman, K. (2014, June 24). *Katy says podcast: Episode 1: Let's talk alignment!* [Audio podcast]. Retrieved from nutritiousmovement.com/podcast-transcript-ep-1-lets-talk-alignment

8. Bowman, K. (2014). *Move your DNA: Restore health through natural movement.* Carlsborg, WA: Propriometrics Press.

9. Romanov, N. (2008). *Pose Method® of triathlon techniques: Become the best triathlete you can be: 3 Sports - 1 Method.* Coral Gables, FL: Pose Tech Press™.

10. Dreyer, D. (2009, Feb. 23). *How to avoid heel strike: Video instruction by Chi Running's Danny Dreyer* [Video file]. Retrieved from www.youtube.com/watch?v=rkUqkdPQHis

Chapter 7

1. Egoscue University®. (2007). EM 201 Posture identification course. San Diego, CA: Egoscue University®.

2. Cherry, K. (2016, June 14). Albert Bandura biography: His life, work and theories. Retrieved from www.verywell.com/albert-bandura-biography-1925-2795537

3. Egoscue, P. (1998). *Pain free: A revolutionary method for stopping chronic pain.* New York, NY: Bantam Books.

4. Heller, M. (2012, June 17). Changing inhibition patterns: Breaking the pain - inhibition - instability cycle. *Dynamic Chiropractic, 30*(13). Retrieved from www.dynamicchiropractic.com/mpacms/dc/article.php?id=55943

Chapter 8

1. Egoscue University®. (2007). EM 201 Posture identification course. San Diego, CA: Egoscue University®.

2. Baechle, T. R. & Earle, R. W. (Eds.). (2000). *Essentials of strength training and conditioning: National strength and conditioning association* (2nd ed.). Champaign, IL: Human Kinetics.

3. Postural Restoration Institute® (PRI). (2015). *Pelvis restoration course: An integrated approach to treatment of patterned pubo-sacral pathomechanics.* Lincoln, NE: Postural Restoration Institute® (PRI).

4. Hruska, R. & Arthur, M. (2013). *Postural Restoration: A new tool for the coaching tool box* [Video file]. Retrieved from www.nsca.com/videos/conference_lectures/postural_restoration_a_new_tool_for_the_coaching_tool_box

5. Egoscue, P. (1998). *Pain free: A revolutionary method for stopping chronic pain.* New York, NY: Bantam Books.

6. Bryant, C. X. & Green, D. J. (Eds.). (2010). *ACE personal trainer manual: The ultimate resource for fitness professionals* (4th ed.). San Diego, CA: American Council on Exercise.

7. Postural Restoration Institute® (PRI). (2016). *Impingement & instability course.* Lincoln, NE: Postural Restoration Institute® (PRI).

Chapter 9

1. Wiebe, J. (2014). *The pelvic floor piston: Foundation for fitness* [Online course]. Retrieved from www.juliewiebept.com/product/the-pelvic-floor-piston-foundation-for-fitness-2

2. Postural Restoration Institute® (PRI). (2015). *Pelvis restoration course: An integrated approach to treatment of patterned pubo-sacral pathomechanics.* Lincoln, NE: Postural Restoration Institute® (PRI).

3. Kendall, F., McCreary, E., Provance, P., Rodgers, M. & Romani, W. (2005). *Muscles: Testing and function with posture and pain* (5th ed.). Baltimore, MD: Lippincott Williams & Wilkins.

4. INTIMINA. (2014, May 14). Dr. Kegel – Pelvic health hero! Retrieved from www.intimina.com/blog/dr-kegel

5. Postural Restoration Institute® (PRI). (2015). *Cervical revolution course: An integrated approach to treatment of patterned cervical pathomechanics.* Lincoln, NE: Postural Restoration Institute® (PRI).

6. Wiebe, J. (2012, June 3). *The core machine: Gears gotta move* [Video file]. Retrieved from www.youtube.com/watch?v=sGykBblgTgU

7. Egoscue University®. (2007). EM 205 Introduction to menu writing course. San Diego, CA: Egoscue University®.

8. Porter, K. (2013). *Natural posture for pain-free living: The practice of mindful alignment.* Rochester, VT: Healing Arts Press.

Chapter 10

1. Postural Restoration Institute® (PRI). (2015). *Pelvis restoration course: An integrated approach to treatment of patterned pubo-sacral pathomechanics.* Lincoln, NE: Postural Restoration Institute® (PRI).

2. Postural Restoration Institute® (PRI). (2014). *Myokinematic restoration course: An integrated approach to treatment of patterned lumbo-pelvic-femoral pathomechanics.* Lincoln, NE: Postural Restoration Institute® (PRI).

3. Kendall, F., McCreary, E., Provance, P., Rodgers, M. & Romani, W. (2005). *Muscles: Testing and function with posture and pain* (5th ed.). Baltimore, MD: Lippincott Williams & Wilkins.

4. Brown, A. (2014, April 28). How many breaths do you take each day? Retrieved from blog.epa.gov/blog/2014/04/how-many-breaths-do-you-take-each-day

5. Masek, J. (2015). Femoroacetabular impingement: Mechanisms, diagnosis and treatment options using Postural Restoration®: Part 2. *SportEX Medicine Journal, 65,* 18-24.

6. Hadfield, J. (2016, July 13). Four ways to stop the dreaded side stitch: You can start by watching what you eat before a run. *Runner's World.* Retrieved from www.runnersworld.com/ask-coach-jenny/four-ways-to-stop-the-dreaded-side-stitch

7. Bradley, B. (2012, July 17). *The Egoscue tower* [Video file]. Retrieved from www.youtube.com/watch?v=HAXaZ0xLWJg

8. Myers, T. W. (2014). *Fascia in movement webinar series* [Webinar]. Retrieved from www.anatomytrains.com/product/fascia-in-movement-webinar-series

9. Postural Restoration Institute® (PRI). (2015). *PRI integration for fitness and movement course: Restoring tri-planar performance through respiration and alternating reciprocal activity.* Lincoln, NE: Postural Restoration Institute® (PRI).

10. Postural Restoration Institute® (PRI). (2014). *Postural respiration course: An integrated approach to treatment of patterned thoraco-abdominal pathomechanics.* Lincoln, NE: Postural Restoration Institute® (PRI).

11. Bartels, L. (n.d.). Postural priorities - Rib cage influences on the volleyball player's shoulder [PDF file]. Retrieved from www.posturalrestoration.com/_resources/e30d:mpdigx-13/files/1061913z50f98e9c/_fn/Postural_Priorities_1.pdf

12. Cantrell, M. (2011). A PRI analytical overview of functional thoracic positioning and thoracic-scapular stability [PDF file]. Postural Restoration Institute®. Retrieved from www.posturalrestoration.com/_resources/e30d:mpd6r1-12/files/1061690za751213/_fn/A_PRI_Analytical_Overview_Of_Functional_Thoracic_Positioning_and_Thoracic-Scapular_Stability.pdf

13. Benson, H. (1975). *The relaxation response.* New York, NY: HarperTorch™.

14. Rankin, L. (2013). *Mind over medicine: Scientific proof that you can heal yourself.* Carlsbad, CA: Hay House, Inc.

15. Stordahl, L. (2012). Why do dogs shake themselves? - The dog 'Body Shake.' Retrieved from www.thatmutt.com/2012/03/08/the-dog-body-shake-why-does-my-dog-shake-his-body

16. Louw, A. (2013). *Why do I hurt?: A patient book about the neuroscience of pain.* Story City, IA: International Spine and Pain Institute.

Chapter 11

1. Hanna, T. (1988). *Somatics: Reawakening the mind's control of movement, flexibility and health.* Cambridge, MA: Da Capo Press.

2. Pfaffmann, C. (2017). Human sensory reception. In *Encyclopaedia Britannica online.* Retrieved from www.britannica.com/science/human-sensory-reception

3. Williamson, C. (2007). *Muscular retraining for pain-free living: A practical approach to eliminating chronic back pain, tendonitis, neck and shoulder tension, and repetitive injuries.* Boston, MA: Trumpeter Books.

4. Vineyard, M. (2007). *How you stand, how you move, how you live: Learning the Alexander Technique to explore your mind-body connection and achieve self-mastery.* Cambridge, MA: De Capo Press.

5. The complete guide to the Alexander Technique. (n.d.). What is the Alexander Technique? What are the benefits of lessons or classes? Retrieved from www.alexandertechnique.com/at.htm

6. Feldenkrais Guild. (2014, Oct. 16). *What is the Feldenkrais Method?* [Video file]. Retrieved from www.youtube.com/watch?v=-GD28QBKyNU

7. Postural Restoration Institute® (PRI), www.posturalrestoration.com, 5255 R Street, Lincoln, NE 68504, (402) 467-4111.

8. Postural Restoration Institute® (PRI). (2015). *Postural visual integration course.* Lincoln, NE: Postural Restoration Institute® (PRI).

9. Postural Restoration Integration Multidisciplinary Engaged (PRIME™) program at the Hruska Clinic™, www.hruskaclinic.com/services/prime.html, 5241 R Street, Lincoln, NE 68504, (402) 467-4545.

10. PRI Vision™ Center, www.privisioncenter.com, 5241 R Street #3, Lincoln, NE 68504, (402) 261-6793.

11. Postural Restoration Institute® (PRI). (2015). *Introduction to PRI and the patterned human body. PRI integration for fitness and movement course: Restoring tri-planar performance through respiration and alternating reciprocal activity.* Lincoln, NE: Postural Restoration Institute® (PRI).

12. Konnikova, M. (2013). The man who couldn't speak and how he revolutionized psychology. *Scientific American*™. Retrieved from blogs.scientificamerican.com/literally-psyched/the-man-who-couldnt-speakand-how-he-revolutionized-psychology

13. Corballis, M. C. (2014, Jan. 21). Left brain, right brain: Facts and fantasies. *PLoS Biol, 12*(1). doi.org/10.1371/journal.pbio.1001767

14. Postural Restoration Institute® (PRI). (2015). *Cervical revolution course: An integrated approach to treatment of patterned cervical pathomechanics.* Lincoln, NE: Postural Restoration Institute® (PRI).

15. Postural Restoration Institute® (PRI). (2016). *Impingement & instability course.* Lincoln, NE: Postural Restoration Institute® (PRI).

16. Glastier, J. (2012). Temperomandibular dysfunction and systemic distress. *International Dentistry – African Edition, 2*(1), 76-80.

Chapter 12

1. Egoscue University®. (2007). EM 206 Application to sports course. San Diego, CA: Egoscue University®.

2. Gambetta, V. & Gray, G. (2002). Implementing functional training and rehab involves challenging conventional regimens and focusing on the body's biomechanical movements. (Excerpt from: *The Gambetta Method: Common sense training for athletic performance*, 1998).

3. Boyle, M. (2004). *Functional training for sports: Superior conditioning for today's athlete.* Champaign, IL: Human Kinetics.

4. Cook, G. (2003). *Athletic body in balance: Optimal movement skills and conditioning for performance.* Champaign, IL: Human Kinetics.

5. Egoscue University®. (2007). EM 205 Introduction to menu writing course. San Diego, CA: Egoscue University®.

6. Wirhed, R. (2006). *Athletic ability and the anatomy of motion* (3rd ed.). New York, NY: Mosby.

7. Gray Institute®, www.grayinstitute.com, 5353 West US 223 Suite B, Adrian, MI 49221, (517) 266-4653.

8. Hruska, R. & Arthur, M. (2013). *Postural Restoration: A new tool for the coaching tool box* [Video file]. Retrieved from www.nsca.com/videos/conference_lectures/ postural_restoration_a_new_tool_for_the_coaching_tool_box

9. Harris, L. (2014, Apr. 10). *PRI squat teaching progression* [Video file]. Retrieved from www.youtube.com/watch?v=YUFXP4qF2MM

10. Patch Fitness®, www.egoscue.com/patchfitness, 12230 El Camino Real #110, San Diego, CA 92130, (800) 933-9811.

11. Patch Fitness®, (n.d.). *The Patch: PatchFitness manual: 100% natural fitness*. San Diego, CA: Patch Fitness®.

12. Bouchette, E. (2008, May 16). Steelers OK Polamalu's alternative training plans. *Pittsburgh Post-Gazette*. Retrieved from www.post-gazette.com/sports/steelers/2008/05/16/ steelers-ok-polamalu-s-alternative-training-plans/200805160133

Chapter 13

1. Starks, R. (2012). Preparing yourself for the unconventional interview. Retrieved from careertipster.com/careerdev/interviewadvice/ preparing-yourself-for-the-unconventional-interview

2. Csikszentmihalyi, M. (1991). *FLOW: The psychology of optimal experience.* New York, NY: HarperPerennial.

3. Wilson, L. (2015, Feb. 9). Famous words from sports figures about competition. Retrieved from www.positiveperformancetraining.com/ famous-words-sports-figures-competition

4. Palmer, R. (2006). *Zone mind, zone body: How to break through to new levels of fitness and performance - by doing less!* Penryn, Cornwall, UK: Ecademy Press.

5. Loehr, J. & Schwartz, T. (2003). *The power of full engagement: Managing energy, not time, is the key to high performance and personal renewal.* New York, NY: The Free Press.

6. Loehr, J. E. (1995). *The new toughness training for sports: Mental, emotional, and physical conditioning from one of the world's premier sports psychologists.* New York, NY: Plume.

7. Arloski, M. (2007). *Wellness coaching for lasting lifestyle change.* Duluth, MN: Whole Person Associates, Inc.

8. Baechle, T. R. & Earle, R. W. (Eds.). (2000). *Essentials of strength training and conditioning: National strength and conditioning association* (2nd ed.). Champaign, IL: Human Kinetics.

9. Friel, J. (2000). *The mountain biker's training bible.* Boulder, CO: VeloPress.

10. Neithercott, T. (2014, February). A fourth Olympics for skier Kris Freeman: Cross-country star fine-tunes his diabetes management for Sochi. *Diabetes Forecast: The Healthy Living Magazine.* Retrieved from www.diabetesforecast.org/2014/feb/behind-the-scenes-with-skier.html

11. Wilma Rudolph biography. Biography.com. Retrieved from www.biography.com/people/wilma-rudolph-9466552

12. Amy Van Dyken. Colorado sports hall of fame. Retrieved from www.coloradosports.org/index.php/who-s-in-the-hall/inductees/item/221-amy-van-dyken.

13. Crouse, K. (2015, June 19). U.S. Open 2015: Mood turns serious after Jason Day's health scare. *The New York Times.* Retrieved from www.nytimes.com/2015/06/20/sports/golf/us-open-2015-mood-turns-serious-after-jason-days-health-scare.html

14. Official world golf ranking. Retrieved from www.owgr.com/ranking

15. Osbourne, R. (n.d.). Exercise efficiency. Measure body fat or strength to weight ratio? Retrieved from www.collegesportsscholarships.com/body-fat-strength-weight-ratio.htm

16. Lohman, T. G. (1992). *Advances in body composition assessment.* Champaign, IL: Human Kinetics Publishers.

17. Esmat, T. (2016, Oct. 7). Measuring and evaluating body composition. Retrieved from www.acsm.org/public-information/articles/2012/01/12/measuring-and-evaluating-body-composition

18. Clark, N. (2013). *Nancy Clark's sports nutrition guidebook: The #1 nutrition resource for active people* (5th ed.). Champaign, IL: Human Kinetics.

Chapter 14

1. The Gremlin-Taming® Institute, www.tamingyourgremlin.com, 7424 Greenville Ave. Suite 113, Dallas, TX 75231, (800) 253-9269.

2. Carson, R. (2003). *Taming your gremlin®: A surprisingly simple method for getting out of your own way.* New York, NY: Quill.

3. Baechle, T. R. & Earle, R. W. (Eds.). (2000). *Essentials of strength training and conditioning: National strength and conditioning association* (2nd ed.). Champaign, IL: Human Kinetics.

4. Rountree, S. (2011). *The athlete's guide to recovery: Rest, relax and restore for peak performance.* Boulder, CO: VeloPress.

5. Loehr, J. & Schwartz, T. (2001). The making of a corporate athlete. *Harvard Business Review, 176,* 120-128.

6. Ballou, J. (2011). Motor skill development. *Instructor to Instructor: The Journal of the Rocky Mountain Professional Ski and Snowboard Instructor, 12-13.*

7. Gallwey, T. & Kriegel, B. (1977). *Inner skiing: The dynamic new approach to mastering the slopes through body/mind awareness.* New York, NY: Bantam Books.

8. Lynch, J. & Scott, W. (1999). *Running within: A guide to mastering the body-mind-spirit connection for ultimate training and racing.* Champaign, IL: Human Kinetics.

Chapter 15

1. Williams, J. (Ed.). (2009). *Applied sport psychology: Personal growth to peak performance* (6th ed.). New York, NY: McGraw-Hill Education.

2. Podlog, L. & Eklund, R. (2006). A longitudinal investigation of competitive athletes' return to sport following serious injury. *Journal of Applied Sports Psychology, 18*(1), 44-68.

3. Frankl, V. E. (2006). *Man's search for meaning: An introduction to Logotherapy.* Boston, MA: Beacon Press.

4. Wilkinson, L. (2017). About Laura Wilkinson. Retrieved from laurawilkinson.com/about

5. Aesop. (2000). *The tortoise and the hare.* Retrieved from www.storyarts.org/library/aesops/stories/tortoise.html

Index

Overtime

*Extend your athletic clock and add points to your
scorecard by executing bonus game-plays!*

Connect with The Pain Free Athlete online to access

FREE *Winning the Injury Game* companion materials:

Self-Assessments	rate your athletic readiness
Videos	practice alignment techniques and strengthening movements
Blogs	read the latest trends in posture, injury prevention, training and conditioning, pain management, and wellness and healing

www.thepfathlete.com

The Pain Free Athlete

Stay in the game for life

357

About the Author

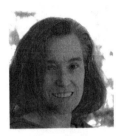

Jessica Kisiel, MS, is The Pain Free Athlete.
Coach, author, and former professional athlete, she is
passionate about the healing capacity of the body and
helps people overcome limitations and pain—so they can
play for the long-term. She holds certifications from the
Postural Restoration Institute® (PRI), Egoscue University®,
National Strength and Conditioning Association (NSCA),
American College of Sports Medicine (ACSM), Wellcoaches
Corporation, and the American Council on Exercise (ACE).
Jessica lives in Moab, Utah.

CPSIA information can be obtained
at www.ICGtesting.com
Printed in the USA
FFOW01n0423050118
44284408-43857FF

9 780999 442500